The Attachment Disability Handbook

The Attachment Disability Handbook

An Introduction and Guide for Counselors, Teachers, and Therapists

John Curran, MD, ABPN

Bidwell Learning Institute

The information in this book is presented for educational purposes. It is not intended to substitute for treatment by a psychotherapist or psychiatrist.

Design by Meadowlark Publishing Services.

Front cover photo © Shutterstock.com/Jacob_09

Published by Bidwell Learning Institute
8014 Olson Memorial Highway
Box 452
Golden Valley, MN 55427
www.attachmentdisability.com

Manufactured in the United States of America.
ISBN 978-0-9996028-1-2

Published 2020

Contents

Introduction

The Attachment Disability Handbook is a distillation of the concepts I developed in *Attachment Disability Volume 1: The Hidden Cause of Adolescent Dysfunction and Lifelong Underperformance.* That book, written primarily for an audience of psychiatrists and psychotherapists, identified Attachment Disability as the residual effects of trauma related to loss, abuse, or neglect in relationships, and as the underlying cause of several conditions that are often misdiagnosed as various forms of mental/emotional disorders. I explained that Attachment Disability may present in three cardinal ways: Attachment Avoidance, Attachment Entanglement, and Attachment Acting-Out.

The concept of attachment was developed by two British psychoanalysts and child psychiatrists, John Bowlby and Donald Winnicott, based on their observations of children and adolescents raised in foster homes, in orphanages, or by biological relatives during the turmoil of World War II. Their notions regarding attachment impairment and its later consequences were a prominent feature of my psychiatric training in the 1960s. My furtherance of their ideas evolved over decades of practice in a variety of settings, including specialty training at the New York State Psychiatric Institute; clinical, research, and consulting work at Minnesota's Anoka State Hospital and Lakeland Mental Health Clinic; serving as a consultant to a dropout program; and extensive office practice.

The very good news about Attachment Disability is that once you identify it, you can manage it through a three-step process I described in the first book, with resulting improvements in quality of life. That's why I created this abbreviated version with the aim of introducing this process to a far wider audience: teachers, counselors, social workers, health care workers, parents and guardians, and others who are in positions to help Attachment Disability sufferers navigate their condition, and ultimately learn to manage it well enough to experience significant relief.

While this book simplifies what I wrote in *Attachment Disability Volume 1*, it contains the core knowledge you will need in order to be of genuine assistance. I have eliminated same case studies that were discursive and obscure while modifying others to clarify their messages. Further, I have discarded the extensive and detailed endnotes and footnotes, here including only footnotes that reference the parent volume—now available as an e-book—for readers whose curiosity leads them to explore certain concepts further. On the other hand, I have retained the essence of its chapters on anxiety and depression, which assert that all anxiety is related to the prospect of separation and abandonment, and that most so-called "depression" is actually cognitive, not emotional: it is self-blame for the paralysis or impulsiveness caused by unrecognized anxiety. In lieu of an index, each chapter now contains a summary of key instructions and guidelines. Moreover, I have collected all of the chapter summaries into a separate PDF file that you can download for easy reference from the Attachment Disability website: www. attachmentdisability.com.

How to Use This Book

The Attachment Disability Handbook consists of two Parts. In Part I, Varieties of Attachment Disability, the three forms of the condition are described, with one chapter devoted to each. Part II, Managing Attachment Disability, begins with a chapter on the strategy and tactics of management. The remaining three chapters of this Part cover the three steps of management: clarifying the condition, learning to accept it, and focusing on what the afflicted individual can change in their behaviors to improve their life experience.

I encourage you to read the chapters in order, as understanding builds from chapter to chapter. But before you start at the beginning, you might want to flip to the end and skim through chapter 7. This will acquaint you with how management of Attachment Disability works in practice as individuals learn to manage their condition. In other words, it will afford you a glimpse of where you are headed after developing a base of knowledge about what Attachment Disability is and the steps involved in easing its effects.

Recent Discoveries

My practice has changed since writing the first volume: I see fewer children and younger adolescents and more older adolescents, young adults, adults, and seniors. This more extensive and in-depth contact across the age spectrum has simply confirmed my belief—as expressed in the term *lifelong underperformance* in the subtitle of the original book—that the reverberation of trauma knows no age constraint. You don't "get over" trauma; you learn how to accept and live with it. So as you peruse these pages, please keep in mind that the concepts I developed years ago with children and adolescents in mind apply to all trauma sufferers.

The change in my practice has brought with it more exposure to individuals with the physical disabilities that accompany the degenerative changes of aging, especially chronic pain. It has become clear to me that the dependency and helplessness that result from the progression of chronic illness unmask and fuel the return of attachment issues that sufferers had previously managed by being active and productive. The ghosts of trauma return to haunt the aging disabled, and fears of abandonment flourish. I believe the insights herein are especially relevant to the understanding and management of these older sufferers.

A Final Note

The alert reader will note a tendency to redundancy in this handbook. When you do, I applaud your alertness and scrutiny because it means you have read the material closely. But I make no apology—this repetition is by design. Both the learning and unlearning of Attachment Disability are generated by repetition, so your appreciation of it is evidence of learning.

May this handbook serve you and those you counsel well.

Part I

Varieties of Attachment Disability

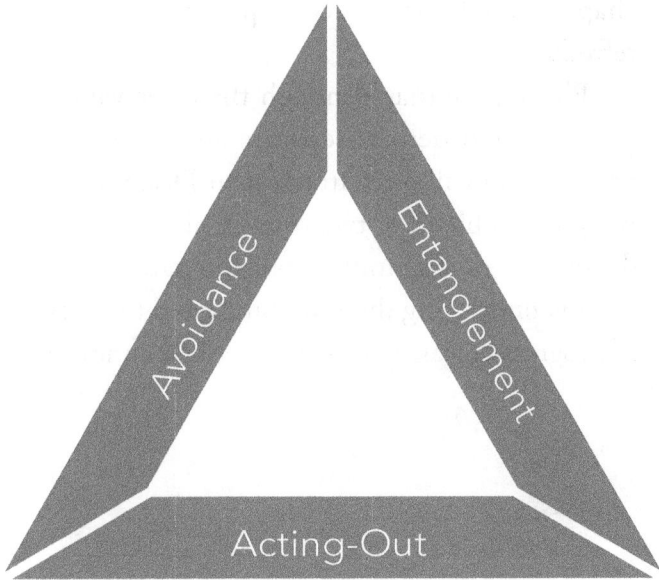

Welcome to Part I of *The Attachment Disability Handbook.* Here you will learn the characteristics of the three varieties of Attachment Disability and how to recognize them in the individuals you work with. Each of the three chapters in this section includes case studies to illustrate the particular type of disability. Each concludes with a bullet-list summary of the main points of the chapter, to reinforce its concepts and for an easy refresher.

Please note that although the three varieties are presented here as separate and distinct, in practice you will find Attachment Disability can present as a blend of two or even all three types, depending on the individual, the nature of the trauma underlying their disability, and their level of progress in learning to manage their condition.

1

Attachment Disability #1: Attachment Avoidance

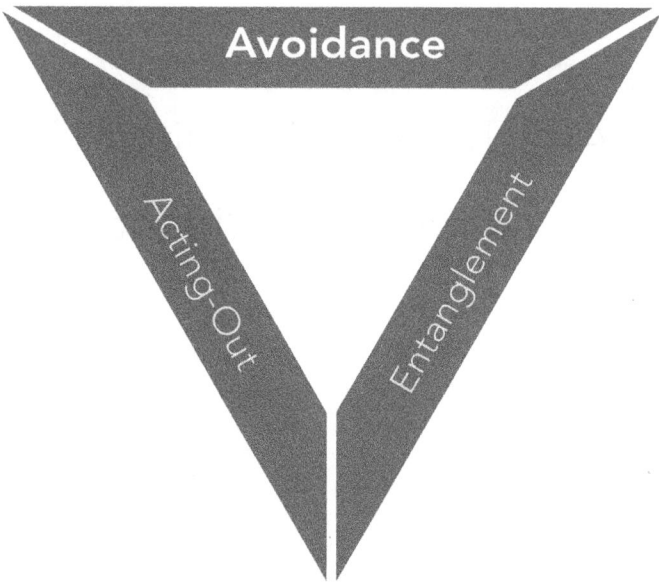

Attachment Avoidance Defined

With this form of Attachment Disability, a lost relationship damages trust so profoundly that trauma survivors are unable to reach out and establish new relationships for fear of being hurt again. Healing stalls out. Life grinds to a halt. School or work performance decays. The person tunnels underground emotionally, becomes closed up and withdrawn, spurns offers of friendship. Survivors may experience panic or anger, radiate despair or apathy, perhaps turn to drugs. Eventually friends and family become impatient with them, clear in their expectation that the suffering loved one should just "get over it."

For their part, sufferers are just as impatient and disgusted with themselves. They feel weak and are unable to explain why they can't get better. Withdrawal and hiding seem to be the only available options.

Those with this form of Attachment Disability are rarely suicidal but sometimes wish they were dead. That would bring peace.

Case Study: Dyllen

"I'm having a lot of anxiety," twenty-two-year-old Dyllen tells me, "and I finally decided I should see somebody about it."

He tells me he has never seen a psychiatrist before, but he can't think what else to do. "How long has anxiety been a problem?" I ask.

"Since I started smoking less pot and drinking less. About a year ago, I started cutting way back on both after using for years. I haven't had anything at all for four months. But it's hard because I get so anxious sometimes. Panic attacks too, and that's just hell."

I note Dyllen's appearance: casually dressed in clean but worn clothing, a fairly attractive young man. His demeanor is attentive, cooperative, compliant; he waits for me to ask questions before offering information. He is also clearly restless, on edge. And I detect undertones of shame as he chronicles his substance use. But there is no blame, of himself or others.

"How do you experience anxiety? What happens?"

"Well, it's gotten so I don't want to leave my apartment. I shop at night, when fewer people will be looking at me—I'm always worrying what other people are thinking about me. The worst is when I'm standing at the checkout and it seems everybody behind me is watching everything I do and I'm just stuck there."

Dyllen gradually picks up steam as we talk, needing fewer prompts to chronicle his disability. I learn that he's been thinking about dying lately; he is quick to assure me he would never commit suicide, but wonders why he would be starting to obsess about his own death. His chronic insomnia is getting worse. He has strange dreams in which someone is in trouble—never anyone he knows—and he's helpless to do anything about it.

When his monologue winds down, I probe further. "Aside from being in your apartment, where are you most comfortable?"

"I'm usually okay at work. I'm a mechanic with a dirt track team. I'm good at it, so they pretty much leave me alone. I can handle the job on my own."

"Did you ever have panic attacks before you started cutting back on marijuana and alcohol?"

"Yeah. The first time was when I was nine. The teacher asked me to get up in front of the class and recite. I was so scared of that, and I just couldn't make myself do it. I was shaking and sweating and everything. I told her no, I wouldn't, and when she got mad and told me a second time to go up there, I started crying. I was only a little kid and I just lost it. And the whole class laughed at me.

"Finally she gave up and made somebody else stand up instead." He pauses, reflecting for a moment, then resumes. "All through school after that I figured out some way to get out of talking in front of people. I'd goof around, or pretend I didn't hear or that I didn't know the answer when I really did. I wasn't ever going to let that happen again if I could help it."

Dyllen is forthcoming about his family history, some

of which is painful. An alcoholic father; loud, violent fights between his father and mother. His mother finally leaving the father and raising Dyllen and his older brother together for a short while by herself. The two siblings got along well, so that was good, but his brother moved out of the house as soon as he could and joined the army.

"That was a shock," he tells me. "Things were better with him around. Living with my mom was mostly okay, but not as good with my brother gone. I liked hanging out with him. He gave me advice, and he helped me sometimes."

"How about later, when you got into high school? How did you do then? Did you like it?"

"I dropped out when I turned sixteen to take a job—that's how I did. No, I didn't like it. I always did well in class but I never did any homework. I didn't get held back, but that dragged my grades down pretty far. Saw a counselor about it once but that never went anywhere. To be honest, for me high school was mostly about smoking pot with my buddies, sneaking beers when we could."

"What job did you take when you dropped out?"

"Auto parts store, stocking parts. I studied the manufacturers' websites more than I ever studied anything in school, and I learned fast—I really am smart when I apply myself, like my mom always said when she was trying to get me to study. I became their go-to guy for off-the-wall questions the clerks couldn't handle. But then the manager wanted me to work up front more, and I quit. From there it was odd jobs and then working on cars for friends and neighbors. Got good at it, so I'm still doing mechanics."

At the end of the session we talk about medication and I write a prescription for a medication that's helpful with social anxiety and insomnia.

"I hope this takes the edge off," Dyllen says.

"I hope so too," I tell him.

Recognizing the Signs in Dyllen

What clues do we have here that Dyllen is struggling with the avoidance type of Attachment Disability? There are a few.

Underperforming

I have seen a lot of young men like Dyllen in my practice: men who are clearly bright, with skills and aptitude, but who drift along, dropping out of school, uprooting budding job prospects, and otherwise not living up to their potential.

In Dyllen's case, I saw a direct link between his first panic attack and the intense abandonment he had already experienced at such a young age: a father lost to alcohol, a mother diverted into battles with the father, and then his most valued companion, his brother, abruptly leaving the household. Confronted in elementary school with a request to change from passive observer to active participant—to become the observed one—he had a severe bout of performance anxiety. And when he responded so visibly and physically in front of his peers, in his mind he faced their disapproval and derision: in other words, even more separation from others, even more loss.

From that point, he sought to avoid a repeat performance, and rather ingeniously became practiced at avoidant behaviors. And the ones he tried and came to rely on—clowning around, playing dumb, and acting stubborn—had the opposite effect of his meltdown at age nine: they earned him the respect of his peers. Thus Dyllen began to chart his course for lifelong underachievement, trading off advancement and opportunity for avoiding the risk of judgment.

There is a particularly thorny dimension to the avoidance strategy: these individuals get good at being invisible. In becoming practiced at the kinds of behaviors that achieve this result, they render themselves colorless and, as such, unlikely to attract the attention of anyone in a position to perceive their suffering and offer to help.

So the problem festered. In Dyllen's case, his anxieties widened and he imagined himself judged by everyone: teachers, neighbors, relatives, even complete strangers. Sometimes the thought popped into his head that when people looked at him—even a casual glance from a stranger—they knew what he was thinking. He knew that was a crazy idea, but he still ruminated on it every time he left the house.

The "Solution" of Addiction

Dyllen found an escape route early, in alcohol and pot. He quickly came to prefer pot, partly because it was cheaper, and easier for a teenager to get. But more than that, he was determined to not turn out like his father, an angry and violent drunk. For him, pot was more of a social escape. He found the other smokers in his midst and made a few good friends. He enjoyed mellowing out with his buddies and feeling his anxieties ebb away.

His motivation faded away as well, though—common among heavy pot smokers in my experience. At school he did well on tests at first because he was a good listener in class and had a strong memory. But he didn't turn in his assignments. His teachers argued that he had good potential, and that if he got after his homework he could do well, but their attention only made him uncomfortable. Ignoring his homework wasn't a deliberate plan, but in the back of his mind it was a way of keeping the heat off—the heat of raised expectations.

The Threat of Help

Dyllen described to me his interactions with the counselor in high school in some detail, and it became clear how confusing the experience was for him.

"Why do you think your work with the school counselor didn't go anywhere?" I ask.

"Oh, I don't know. It was just weird. I remember thinking she was just going to tell me to shape up like everybody else was telling me, and I'd have to listen to that for a whole hour. But she was really nice, and it seemed like she was really interested in me, and she asked me a bunch of questions—like you're doing right now, now that I think about it. But I think I wasn't ready for it then."

"Any ideas about why you weren't ready?"

"I was used to getting yelled at about school by my mom, and even by my brother after a while. That was normal. Asking me what was going on with me was *not* normal. I remember being at a complete loss for what to say because I didn't want to tell her how I felt—or why I was doing what I was doing. Partly, I was confused about it all, so I didn't really know myself, but I also knew I was hurting somehow, deep down. Plus, it was weird—even though I'd just met her, I remember thinking I didn't want her to worry about me. Doesn't make a lot of sense, looking back on it."

"So what did you say?"

"Not much, I don't think. She wound up doing most of the talking, about my potential and what-not. Same old song but maybe just … kinder about it, less blame-y. She talked about a discussion group I could join that she thought would be good for me—me, the guy who never wanted to talk in front of class. That was never going to fly."

"So where did you leave things with her?"

"At the end she said she liked meeting me and thought she could help. She invited me back and I told her I'd think about it. That was a straight-up lie though, and she probably knew it—the whole thing made me feel squirmy. She tried calling my mother to have her talk me into it, but I just didn't want to."

"And that was your last counseling session, until this one, what, seven, eight years later?"

"Yeah, that was it."

Dyllen falls silent, seeming to have finished with the topic. Then he offers, "I did get one thing out of it, though. That counselor was the one who pointed out to me how far behind I was, because she had all my grades, the big picture. She told me I was too far behind to be able to graduate without repeating a grade. And you know what? I felt relieved. It felt like then I had permission to bail. I started cutting school—a lot. But then a truancy officer got involved and told my mom we'd have to go to court, and there was another time when my mom just freaked out about how hard I was making everything for her, like being a single mom isn't hard enough. I felt so guilty that I started attending classes again, but man, I hated it."

His face brightens suddenly. "There was one class I liked, though, a drafting class I took. I guess that makes sense for somebody who's a mechanic now, right? I did well there, but it wasn't enough."

"And so you dropped out at sixteen."

"Yep. By that time my mom had given up—she was just tired of fighting me about it, I think. So when I told her I wanted to drop out right after my birthday, she said fine, but you need to get a job."

The Solution of Work—and the Threat of Success

It didn't take long to discover the highlights in Dyllen's life: success at his auto parts store job, working on cars for his buddies and their friends and families and learning he had a knack for it, then taking that talent into his current job. In his case, I can say that for Dyllen, dropping out of school in favor of work turned out to be an excellent decision. He left a world where he was failing and entered a world that could actually put his interests and aptitudes to good use—and that didn't demand a lot of visibility.

But Dyllen's patterns of behavior followed him into the workplace as well. His boss at the auto parts store offered to promote him, give him more face-to-face contact with customers along with a raise. He also told him that if he went back and got his GED, he could be eligible for a manager's job in a few years at one of the other stores in the chain—salary, benefits, a real step ahead.

All of Dyllen's fears immediately flooded back at the suggestion, and his body rebelled every bit as much as it had when he was nine years old and was being told he had to speak in front of the class. His face flushed, he felt hot—he felt trapped—and all he knew was that he had to escape that conversation. He mumbled something and walked away. His boss had no idea what his employee was experiencing, of course, and took offense, angry at what he saw as insolent rejection of a generous offer. An argument ensued and culminated with Dyllen tossing his cap and his keys on the counter, saying, "I quit!" and walking out.

A series of odd jobs—entailing no threat of commitment or advancement—led him at last to his current job, which seemed like it could work out for him in the long run. That is, he reasoned, even if the dirt track job dried up at some point, there's always a market for car mechanics, and they tend to spend a lot of time working solo, behind the scenes. Unobserved, unchallenged.

Guys who work on cars "get to be left alone," as Dyllen put it to me.

The Mystery of Change

In my limited work with Dyllen, I didn't get the chance to probe how he came to the decision to stop using drugs and alcohol. In my experience it always seems easier to reconstruct why things fall apart than why they improve. I imagined a girlfriend in the mix somehow, someone who became invested in his well-being and eventually asked him why he smoked so much pot, urged him to make some changes there. I envisioned arguments during which he resisted and she retreated, until finally one day she decided she didn't want a pothead for a boyfriend anymore and told him that. Perhaps by that time, Dyllen was invested in her too, and his fundamental dread of separation kicked in.

He started cutting back, and as he did so, the pain he had been suppressing came to the fore. He decided he was going to try to face it—in manageable doses at first, tempered by using when things got too scary. Somehow, he managed to emerge from the haze for long enough stretches of time to see the extent of his pain, the depth of it, and he realized that if he was going to stay clean, he'd need some help in coping with it.

And he found his way to my door.

Dyllen Returns

I'm surprised to see Dyllen when he returns two years later, but he's on a mission and he thinks I can help. It turns out the girlfriend I had posited is real, and she has stood by him, and he's still doing well at the dirt track—in fact, the crew says he's the best mechanic they've ever worked with. But they've also told him he should get his GED so he can go to community college and learn computer programming to keep up with the technology involved. He's not intimidated by that, I learn; computers have become sort of a hobby for him. But as for returning to school, and to the scrutiny of teachers and classmates, the old panicky feelings are back. Can I help him?

He's not asking for a prescription this time. I recommend an anxiety management program so he can "toughen his hide" before reentry into the classroom without having to see a counselor on a regular basis. He likes the idea and tells me that he bets his girlfriend would be up for helping him with it.

I sense that Dyllen will find a way to overcome his performance issues, or if not, at least learn to live with them well enough to proceed with his education. And I hope I won't have to wait too many years to find out how things are going.

Case Study: Holden Caulfield— To Trust Is Dangerous

The next attachment avoidant individual I'd like to introduce you to is a fictional creation, a literary figure who emerges from the pages of J. D. Salinger's *The Catcher in the Rye:* Holden Caulfield. I invite you to consider Holden in the context of this chapter on Attachment Avoidance because in several ways, he perfectly exemplifies the profile of an adolescent spirit grappling with this form of Attachment Disability.

The book's protagonist, Holden is impulsive, bumbling, sensitive, horny, opinionated, compassionate, and grieving. For decades, adolescent readers have come to adopt Holden as the embodiment of lost innocence, of rebellion against corrupt adult authority. But this does him and Salinger a disservice. Rather, Holden struggles to cope with the loss of his beloved younger brother as well as his persisting ambivalence about reaching out for adult support. This is the signature conflict of today's troubled adolescent. *Catcher* was published in 1951, and to my way of thinking Salinger was eerily prophetic: his is a profile of a young man who is conflicted, struggling to risk becoming attached in a world that has been revealed to be painfully unpredictable.

The Backstory

Three years have passed since Holden's eleven-year-old brother, Allie, died from leukemia, yet Holden's wounds remain unhealed. The loving and secure relationship he has lost is still the standard by which all others are measured and found wanting, with the exception of his older brother, D. B.; his younger sister, Phoebe; and his sweetheart, Jane. In fact Holden still talks to Allie "sort of out loud" when he feels depressed.

The night Allie died, Holden slept in the garage. He broke some windows, but clearly more than windows were broken, and not all has been repaired since. Holden is being kicked out of prep school, not because he isn't smart but because he's blocked, which most likely accounts for three prior prep school debacles. Here is an example of how the idealized image of a lost relationship, while comforting, is also paralyzing. Holden remains gripped by what has been lost.

The same is true of his parents, but their sensibilities and personalities are vaguely drawn. Each in his or her own way has withdrawn from Holden, who understands their "touchiness" because of his own misery. So he evades them, sneaking in and out of their apartment on a midnight visit to see Phoebe.

Recognizing the Signs in Holden

Some consider Holden the prototype of teenage rebelliousness. True, he is forever detecting "phoniness" in his world, and few escape his critical eye. However, he does not play the rebel, does not debate or argue or confront or otherwise engage any of these "phony" figures: the hallmark of the rebel.

Withdrawal

Rather, he withdraws. At one point Phoebe asserts that his problem is that he doesn't like anything, and Holden is hard pressed to refute her. His critical spirit is not one of antagonism toward others but protection of himself.

His fantasy is to go on the bum, find a job at a filling station, and pretend to be a deaf-mute: "and then I would be through with having conversation for the rest of my life." Later he would build a cabin in the woods, marry a beautiful deaf-mute, and hide their children. The idea of someone mourning him after death is repellent. He hopes someone "has sense enough to just dump me in the river or something ... Who wants flowers when you are dead?"

Protectiveness

Holden's dream, and the theme of the novel, is his notion of protecting children from harm. As he explains to Phoebe, he would be stationed at the edge of a cliff beside a field of rye in which thousands of kids play unsupervised, with "nobody big" to catch them if they run too close to the edge and fall over: "If they are running and they don't look where they are going I have to come out from somewhere and catch them ... I'd be the catcher in the rye." His hurt is so profound that he dreads the possibility of anyone feeling the pain of separation and loss ... so he avoids.

Eventually protectiveness overrules avoidance when he attempts to persuade Phoebe, who is determined to run away with him out west, to stay home. At first she angrily rejects him, refuses his offer to accompany her back to school, and runs through traffic across the street, where she stops and eyes him. Figuring she will follow him, Holden enters Central Park, where they have spent many afternoons playing. She catches up with him, and after he changes his mind and promises her he won't leave town, she relents somewhat. On their way home they pass the carousel, Phoebe's favorite, still open despite the season. He persuades her to take a ride, she agrees, and suddenly she's no longer mad at him. She kisses him, rides again.

As she rides he gets soaked in an unseasonable winter rain, but he doesn't care because she is so happy going round and round. "I was damn near bawling, I felt so damn happy." Having accepted her gift of the redemptive power of unconditional regard, he has begun to heal, and with this he realizes a fundamental truth about childhood: "The thing with kids is, if they want to grab the gold ring, you have to let them do it, and not say anything. If they fall off they fall off, but it's bad if you say anything to them." He has learned that to be alive is to accept uncertainty and not be trapped by protective feelings toward others. And he is no longer threatened by feelings of joy and happiness.

And it seems he has learned another lesson. He reports he's sorry he's talked so much because he now realizes he misses everyone he's talked about. "It's funny. Don't ever tell anybody anything. If you do, you start missing everybody."[1] Holden senses that to confide is risky because

---

1. It seems Salinger followed Holden's advice. In the years after the book's publication, he became reclusive, retreating to a remote New Hampshire town, never giving an interview, publishing little. One wonders if he later felt he had revealed too much of himself as he constructed Holden's identity; hence his protectiveness.

it establishes intimacy and vulnerability. Be careful, he tells us.

Death Paralyzes

Part of the book's artistry is the subtle manner in which Salinger introduces us to Holden's grief and suffering while precisely capturing the adolescent struggle to cope with loss. Death deflates, stuns, numbs.

Kids (and adults) experiencing Attachment Avoidance wander into my office distracted and diffident, not enraged; they are reluctant or even unable to reveal the shock precipitated by the death of siblings or peers or parents or beloved grandparents. School and work performance decline and may even evaporate.

Holden is aware of the nature of his loss—this is not true of all. With some, a tangible external loss has evolved into an intangible inner loss; that is, they feel they have lost control of their thoughts or feelings or bodies. They have lost security. Only at home, sometimes only in their bedroom, do they feel safe. Their loss, whatever its content, has taken on symbolic qualities. Usually most of the familiar necessities remain—home, family, circle of friends, shelter, food, clothing. All needs appear satisfied. Yet things are different, irrevocably changed. Their tomorrows now appear less inviting.

These individuals often offer very vague explanations for why they are not attending school or working: they just don't want to, it's meaningless, they feel "depressed," and so on. Sometimes they can't sleep; at other times they sleep all the time. Typically they look more anxious than depressed.

Individuals who are less gripped by denial have enough insight to be able to describe the turmoil of their inner world. They talk about unwanted emotions: jealousy, anger, even love. Or distressing repetitive thoughts (obsessions) or behaviors (compulsions). They say their body feels funny or sick: their heart pounds, they can't stop sweating, they are dizzy, they feel walled off from everything; that is, *dissociated.* Typically, they worry that if people knew how they felt or thought, they would be judged weak or immature or helpless. The truth about their inner world would be catastrophic if known to others. *People will withdraw from you and abandon you. Or they will tease you and pick on you. Or, worse yet, they will overwhelm you with help and you will be smothered.*

Even these relatively insightful individuals may have difficulty relating their feeling state to a prior loss, instead shrinking from the obvious connection. It just feels safer to stay home, go to school online. Relationships are less dangerous at a distance. Otherwise they feel as if their identity might dissolve. Turning to alcohol or street drugs to relieve the misery and turmoil is tempting, and many, like Dyllen, do not resist.

Case Study: Helen

I am seeing Helen, a twenty-year-old bioengineering student, following up on how she's doing with the medications I had prescribed for her a few weeks earlier for persistent loneliness, sadness, "depression," and anxiety.

When Helen first came to my office, she presented as an intelligent, well-groomed, cooperative young woman. One of the first things I learned about her was that she had received grief counseling periodically for nearly her entire life, since the age of eight when her mother suddenly died from an undiagnosed sepsis. Antidepressants were only marginally helpful.

"What was your childhood like after your mother died?" I had asked when she shared this with me.

"It was hard," she said. "I had other family, my dad and my brother, but they only seemed to like me if I acted happy. My mom had died—how could I be happy all the time? It was like they wanted me to be a different person."

We moved on to relationships in her present life, and she immediately became tearful. She had clearly reflected on her relationship difficulties a great deal and had some good insights. "I think that first abandonment when I was so little, I think it's affected everything. I've learned to keep my distance. Nobody can abandon you if you're not that close to them in the first place, right?"

Indeed. "So what do you do, exactly, to keep your distance?" I asked.

"I keep to myself. I want to be alone all the time. It feels like I'll be okay as long as I'm alone. I mean, I should say I'll be okay-*ish*—it's kind of like being in limbo. But it's when I'm with other people that I start to feel outright depressed, so I avoid it when I can."

Months later, during Christmas break, Helen returns, having switched psychiatrists in the interim and tried a few other medications. She has also joined a Depression support group, but despite all her efforts, her life has taken a turn for the worse.

"I had to take incompletes in three of my four classes this semester," she says. "I was so … so out of it. I couldn't think straight. I couldn't even get out of bed. I'm scared that life isn't going to get any better than this. I either feel numb or I'm depressed—those seem like my only choices.

"And I know it's my fault, because I isolate myself, but I don't feel supported or wanted anywhere. I just feel alone. Even when I went to visit my best friend—somebody I think of as my best friend, anyway—it seemed like she wasn't all that happy to be spending time with me."

"Let me give you a different way to think about your depression," I suggest. "Next time you think, 'I'm depressed,' instead think, 'I'm feeling fearful.'" (Attachment disabled people often use the term "depressed" as a kind of catchall term for their emotional state when the underlying experience is actually stress, anxiety, worry, or apprehension. For further discussion of this misnomer, see chapter 5 in this handbook and chapters 8 and 9 in *Attachment Disability, Volume 1*.)

Three weeks after that visit, Helen applied for medical leave from school. She packed up her belongings, sublet her apartment, and enrolled in a day treatment program. Under the care of another psychiatrist, she modified her psychotropic regimen yet again. She is now taking a complex cocktail of four different medications.

"Despite all that stuff I'm taking, and all the help I'm getting," she tells me, "I'm *still* depressed—sad, low energy, never hungry, always tired. I've lost ten pounds in the last two months, and I don't have all that much to spare." The only bright spot she can point to is that she has a new job, as a receptionist at a law firm.

"Perhaps you're still dealing with the residual trauma of your mother's death," I suggest, not for the first time.

"Yeah, that's probably always in there somewhere," she admits. "But really, I just don't trust people, and that's depressing. I think people are selfish, always doing what's best for themselves. It always feels like I'm the one who has to bend over backward."

"Well, we can look at that," I offer, "but right now let's address your medication situation. You're on a lot of medications, and they don't seem to be helping. Let's start backing off the dosages—but let's put you in the driver's seat on that. You can be your own doctor, in terms of the sequence and rate of tapering. Just tell me how you want to do it, and I'll let you know if I think you should go slower, for safety. Other than that, let's put you in charge."

This approach offers a way for Helen to achieve a sense of control, of mastery of her own life, and reduces my role to advisor and co-observer of a process she is initiating.

From that point, I saw Helen for lengthier and more frequent visits, about fifteen of them altogether, part medication management and part psychotherapy. We talked about events in her life since the previous visit, her emotional responses to them, and the decisions she'd made. We particularly worked on clarifying her thoughts and feelings and helping her *own the pain in her life without blame* (see chapter 6 for a discussion of this therapeutic goal).

Over the course of those weeks, she began to demonstrate increasing decisiveness. She decided to drop out of the day treatment program she'd been in. She changed grief counselors. She made plans to move out of her parents' place and into her own apartment. She began to connect with a coworker and arranged a coffee date.

"Trusting like that was strange, setting up that weekend coffee date," she tells me. "To think I could maybe be myself with someone that way, that was new. But it actually felt okay."

During another session she described for me what we would both come to see as a pivotal moment for Helen. She had spontaneously decided to assist a bus passenger who was having difficulty navigating his wheelchair while juggling his belongings.

"I forgot about everything when I was doing that. It made me feel good that I did something for someone. It was just a spur-of-the-moment thing, but you know what? I feel the happiest I've felt in months."

During another visit, she tells me of an epiphany she had while working with a grief counselor.

"I realized that it's hard to hear other people talk about my mother, what they experienced with her. I want my memories of her to be mine, just mine, not what other people remember. The problem is, I have so few of them. I was so little when she died."

The next time she reveals a seemingly small thing that holds some significance.

"I've always been totally fussy about my nails, getting them just right, so I do them myself. But I actually went into a nail salon yesterday and turned my hands over to somebody else. That was so unlike me."

"That sounds to me like a sign that you're increasingly able to trust people," I offer.

"Hmm," she responds, pondering. "You could be right about that ..."

The intervals between visits lengthened as Helen began to benefit from neuropsychological training she was receiving and the tapering of medications. She decided to return to school.

Six months later, we checked in by phone.

"School is going well, and I'm getting along with my roommates," she reports. "And I've decided to switch my goals for school. I'm planning on a doctorate in neuroscience now. I feel like I can help more people that way." Perhaps this was how her experience helping the man in the wheelchair was reverberating in her life; she had discovered then that serving others was a mood lifter.

A few years later, Helen is kind enough to invite me to her graduation party. She greets me with a wide smile.

"You look happy, Helen," I say. "Big day for you, isn't it?"

"It's a big day, yes, but I'm often happy these days, just in general. All the work I did with you, my grief counselor, my neuropsychological therapist—a cast of thousands, you might say," she grins. "Well it's finally paying off. I've learned how to reach out to people. Seems almost like a miracle in retrospect, compared to how I was. But the secret was really what you told me one day in your office. I remember it so vividly. You said, 'Your job is to understand what is happening with you and learn to manage it. To be the detective of your life.'

"And you know what I've figured out?" she concluded. "The more you do that, the easier it gets."

Lessons from Helen

There are two points to cover here:

The Persistence of Attachment Disability

There is a common "wisdom" that attachment issues are solely a phenomenon of early childhood. The idea seems to be that children will "get over it." But perhaps that is simply wishful thinking—the same wish that friends and family of attachment avoidant people have when they grow impatient with their loved one's avoidant behavior. Obviously, Helen did not "get over" the death of her mother at age eight. And her family was of little solace because of their expectations of her behavior; that was an additional loss. So not only did Helen not outgrow her attachment issues, but they festered throughout childhood and adolescence and exploded once she left for college.

The Dynamism of Self-Management

It was encouraging at Helen's graduation party to hear that she recalled my advice about the importance of understanding and managing her condition versus diagnosing and treating it. The idea of this strategy for Attachment Avoidance in particular is to maintain awareness of two basic dynamisms that energize the behavior—distrust and vulnerability.

Attachment Disability is a condition for which the typical hierarchical nature of the doctor/patient relationship is not only often ineffective but can be harmful. Teacher/student interaction is better suited to helping people heal. While it is still hierarchical in the sense that the teacher is presumed to be an expert and expected to provide guidance, it is well understood that *the student also has responsibilities.* And in Helen's case, we both came to the same conclusion: she needed *management,* not *treatment,* and she needed to learn how to manage her disability herself by learning what helped and what did not. I will discuss this distinction at greater length in the section on management.

Ultimately, through trial and error based on her own explorations, she found her way.

Your Takeaways

The attachment avoidant person is unable to reach out for fear of being hurt again.

▲

The anxiety resulting from loss can paralyze; withdrawal and hiding are hallmarks of Attachment Avoidance.

▲

Inexplicable sabotage of success is a hallmark of trauma; watch for a decline in school or work performance.

▲

Attachment Avoidance can make failure feel like the only safe haven in a risky world. Relationships create vulnerability.

▲

Healing from loss involves accepting the uncertainty of life.

2

Attachment Disability #2:
Attachment Entanglement

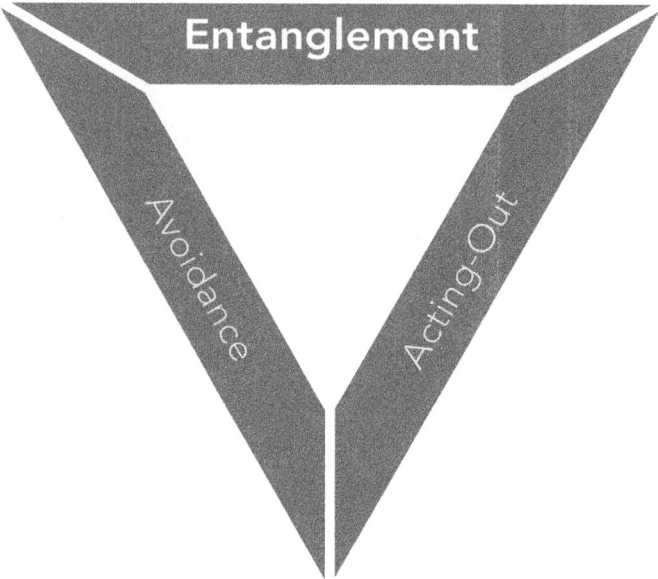

Entanglement

Avoidance

Acting-Out

Attachment Entanglement Defined

Trauma changes a person's sensitivities. A flame or frost burn can permanently alter our ability to endure subsequent exposure to heat or cold. The same is true of the psychological burning of a traumatized relationship. Individuals, young people especially, may be so sensitized by the experience that they become too aware of others' suffering and unhappiness—especially peers and family—and feel increasingly responsible for their welfare. Their appreciation of their own needs and feelings becomes engulfed and smothered—*entangled*—by their perceived sensitivity to the needs and feelings of the other. They often report worrying about "everything." (Therapists describe this attachment style as *enmeshment.*) They have difficulty constructing boundaries, become too immobilized to escape, and sink into a state of emotional paralysis, complaining of "depression." Attachment Entanglement issues can also cause abuse victims to return to an abusive relationship, hoping for one last chance to heal the wounds they perceive are torturing their abuser.

In my experience adolescent girls are more likely than boys to develop this attachment style. If they manage to navigate their adolescent and early adult life without a life disaster, they may be attracted to careers in nurturing professions (medicine, veterinary medicine, teaching, or counseling, for example) and occasionally criminal justice: police or probation officer.

Case Study: Amy

Amy is a college student referred to me from an emergency room, where she had been taken because of suicidal talk. I am to evaluate her, and the ER staff has recommended she enroll in a day treatment program for group therapy and individual counseling. The referral indicates she has been taking an Antidepressant for four months. She has experienced no side effects from the medication—or any benefits.

When she arrives at my office, she is accompanied by her mother. I gesture for Amy to sit down in the usual patient seat, an armchair across a low table from my own chair. I wheel an extra desk chair over for her mother and place it at arm's length from Amy's. When her mother is seated I begin our conversation as I always do, directing my question to Amy. "What brings you here today?"

"They made me come here," she says. "I don't know …" Her voice trails off.

Amy sits defensively, her legs curled up against her and her arms wrapped around them, her eyes cast toward the floor. She looks up briefly and engages a bit with a smile, then breaks eye contact again. I note that she is well groomed, and she seems alert, but she remains silent.

"Have you seen a therapist before?" I ask.

"Yes," she says quietly. "I was seeing someone, once a week, then three times a week the past few weeks. I'm not sure why though …" With the recent frequency of the sessions, there must be good chemistry between them—a hopeful sign, I conclude.

When I prompt her for details, however, she first becomes angry and then tearful. "My medicine doesn't work!" is her response.

Her mother chimes in then. "It's true. We haven't seen much improvement. She's not happy. She doesn't smile. She just gets through the day."

Amy remains huddled and withdrawn as her mother fills in further details. "Things were rough last year at her small college. First a student committed suicide—over-dose—and then two months later another died from bone cancer. It shook up the whole school. Everybody ended the year numb, and when they came back this year they were just plain mad about it all.

"I don't know if that started it, but she recently broke up with her boyfriend too, and there's a clique that's been badmouthing her. She was doing so well before last year—good grades, excelled in athletics. Now she's just ... depressed, anxious, angry."

Amy remains unengaged, and close to tears.

Armed now with information about Amy's previous accomplishments, I realize I've been misinterpreting her restiveness and withdrawal. I've taken them for immaturity, but given her previous record of performance, that no longer fits. *Could the problem be entanglement?* I wonder.

The interview with Amy is clearly going nowhere, so I decide to try another tack. Making use of some stagecraft, I remove my glasses and rub my eyes. "I'm tired," I say. "And we're not getting anywhere. Let's try a different approach."

Donning my lecture persona, I speak at length about "antistressants."[2] I talk about how people avoid intimacy by building barriers through behavior rather than words, and about how vulnerability and fears of trusting might signal entanglement issues.

By mid-discourse, Amy is leaning forward and occasionally smiling. Encouraged, I continue, discussing her vulnerability to sudden self-destructive impulses. I tell her that such behavior indicates she's feeling isolated and guilty, and beginning to feel hopeless.

She says nothing, only nods, but it's clear I've broken through.

---

2. Antidepressants actually work by relieving anxiety and stress, which reduces functional paralysis. Patients become productive, their self-esteem improves, and they like themselves better; hence, "I feel less depressed."

"And that's why they recommended you start a day treatment program, to provide a support system until things are better. It's important that you attend."

She nods again in apparent agreement.

"Your behavior is really different now than it was when you first sat down with me. You know that, right?" I note her more relaxed, open posture—feet on the floor now and hands draped over the armrests—as well as her clear interest in what I am saying.

"Yes," she responds.

"Why is that?"

"I don't know," she shrugs, dropping her eyes.

"Then let me guess. You were afraid to let me get too close—then you'd have someone else to worry about. You already feel a lot of responsibility for everyone."

Amy raises her eyes and meets my gaze directly then, and I know I've hit home.

Recognizing the Signs in Amy

Amy's behavior is a fine illustration of the long-standing psychiatric dictum "You *watch* what patients *say* and *listen* to what they *do*." As her situation unfolded, it began to shout entanglement and thus the need for a less personal relationship, for more distance, which I created by assuming a professorial role.

Pretending Ignorance

Pretending ignorance—"I don't know why they made me come here"; "I don't know why I was in therapy";

"I don't know why my behavior has changed since I got here"—is a form of *resistiveness*. It represents a surrender of responsibility, a silent plea to be treated as a kid, a child in need of protection: *Don't expect too much of me*. This is why I suggest beginning an initial interview with an open-ended, unstructured comment like "Tell me brings you here today." It gives you an opportunity to assess the maturity of the individual before you.

Except for the infrequent situation when you're dealing with an obviously angry individual, I generally would not directly challenge such a pretense of ignorance. Instead you can prod a bit and provide structure in the form of cues that might offer a relatively safe topic for discussion. If that fails, in cases where you suspect entanglement, as was true of Amy, establishing distance can help.

Defensive Posture

Young people present in a variety of ways. Some are elaborately groomed and coiffed, with an attentive posture and expression. Others slouch, or play with a cell phone, or bicker with the adult who accompanies them, or sit rigidly with a defiant expression, or—especially younger ones—roam the office. Amy's posture was unusual in terms of how physically closed off and protective it was; it clearly signified she required careful management.

Greater Comfort with an Impersonal Approach

Earlier I mentioned "stagecraft." By that I mean designing the setting and style of the interview to retain and promote the attentiveness of the person you're interviewing. An attachment-disabled child, adolescent, or adult has difficulty learning—*which is the essential point of therapy*—because they are experiencing "emotional interference." In other words, fear and distrust erode their attentiveness and hence their ability to learn from experience. Stagecraft simply means manipulating the learning venue to retain the learner's attention. Good teachers are performers ... as are good therapists. As a therapist I am always modulating the degree of distance versus intimacy required to enhance attentiveness without smothering it, and that goal is worth the creative effort of engaging in a little "performance art."

So with Amy, I both announced and signaled a change in the interview transaction with a bit of stagecraft designed to create distance by reverting to a format that would be familiar to her student persona: the lecture. The idea was to address the notions of trust and entanglement in a very general fashion, without specifically stating that these might be *her own* personal issues. This left it up to her to decide whether they fit or not. (Further details on stagecraft can be found in *Attachment Disability Volume 1*. See page 267 and the index, especially the need to practice boundary awareness with angry individuals as well.)

Vulnerability to Suicide

Amy's change in posture and smiling attentiveness were signals that the ideas I was floating were a fit. At that point, it seemed safe to personalize things a bit by addressing what her most concerning behavior—talk of suicide—was telling us: that she was isolated, guilty, feeling hopeless. In short, her support system was shaky, which was why attending day treatment was important. Her silent agreement to that suggestion meant that death thoughts, perhaps even suicidal ruminations, had been on her mind, so there was no need to have her confirm this by asking her directly.

Cutting is always a sign of entanglement, "ping-pong" suicidal behavior between peers—where one peer attempts suicide and then another follows suit—an extreme sign.

Overprotectiveness

Amy is an excellent example of how an entangled young person's overprotectiveness can extend to relative strangers. Her concern was that if she told me what she truly felt—for example, guilt and feelings of hopelessness—I would find that upsetting, and then she would have even more to feel guilty about. She didn't need another soul to feel responsible for, to protect. Hence her initial resistiveness and seeming immaturity.

The Mother's Intervention

Amy's case demonstrates the value of including sponsors in the evaluation process, both to flesh out the subject's history and to have the opportunity to observe the sponsor-subject interaction. Typically, unless things have begun with an argument or confrontation, the adults or sponsors in the room do not intervene until I signal for their input. But here, the mother saw that her daughter was floundering and came to her rescue, providing critical information that the daughter could not bear to reveal herself. This suggested Attachment Entanglement guilt was underlying Amy's resistance to engagement.

The Way, Not the Why

What is important in Amy's story is not *why* Amy is the way she is, but confirmation of the *way* she is: entangled. What she needs in order to learn how to manage the anxieties of relationships is an *understanding* of her predicament, not an *explanation*.

Case Study: Charlotte—Shark Attack

"I feel like a fish in a pool full of sharks."

This poignant statement sums up the many reasons Charlotte has come to me seeking anti-anxiety medication. A thirty-three-year-old single mother of two, she has plenty to feel anxious about. She has applied for a job, she's moving, and her abusive partner is about to be released from prison.

When she next returns to see me, she reports that the medication I've prescribed seems to be working. But this relief is short lived. At the following session, she tells me she landed the job she was after—a position as an attendant at a facility for the disabled—but along with it came panic attacks so intense that she had to quit after just two days.

This time Charlotte has returned to my office with instructions from her mother to ask for an Antidepressant. I note the request but shift the conversation to their relationship.

"How do you get along with your mother?"

"Well ..." She thinks for a moment. "Our relationship is pretty intense. We talk every day."

"So you two are close," I suggest.

"Well ... that's one way to put it," she says. Then she throws up her hands. "She controls everything I do!"

She tells me that in fact, that's the reason she decided to move—to get some distance from her mother. "I'm a grown woman, for god's sake," she complains. "I have kids of my own. I can't always be thinking about her."

Over a series of sessions, I learn the origin of "always thinking about her": her mother had been a meth-head when Charlotte was a child. Charlotte had had to care for her mom for literally as long as she could remember.

The fact that it took several sessions for her to reveal her mother's drug dependence told me that she still felt the need to protect "Mom." This need bound her to her mother and would continue to do so indefinitely without some active management of her attachment issues.

Charlotte is a sensitive and empathetic soul, common traits among the entangled. She had continued to endure her mother's "controlling everything I do"—in the form of daily hectoring and fussing—because she had intuited that her mother needed to be needed. She also understood that her mother would experience Charlotte's independence as abandonment, and Charlotte's persistent youthful caretaker persona would find her mother's pain of being left behind intolerable. Thus she remained entangled.

During a session shortly after her mother's addiction came to light, I recall the shark analogy and follow a hunch. "When you were working at the facility, with people who all needed a lot of help, did it feel like every client there wanted a piece of you?"

"Yes!" she replies emphatically.

Recognizing the Signs in Charlotte

It made sense that Charlotte panicked after placing herself in a work environment with people whose needs were never ending. This choice of work is not uncommon for someone raised in an abusive environment; they can become sensitized to suffering and develop a strong sense of empathy. But once on the job, Charlotte was overwhelmed by her clients' needs, felt consumed by them; there would be no end to their calls for help.

Feeling trapped, she panicked, and leapt out of the "pool of sharks." More entanglement would surely be the death of her!

Case Study: Georgina— Parental Entanglement

"Her grades have gone straight downhill," Georgina's mother tells me. "I'm getting worried that if she doesn't turn this around, she won't be accepted to college anywhere."

Georgina sits quietly as her mother describes this recent turn of events. She is a good-looking, mature seventeen-year-old who presents as remote, detached, impassive, composed. I get the sense she is very practiced in affecting this attitude while her mother chronicles her shortcomings.

"I'm sure some of it has to be the pot smoking—she's been hanging out with a bunch of other kids who smoke. How can you focus on your studies when you're getting high all the time?" She spreads her hands, as if to emphasize this question, while looking pointedly at me, apparently hoping to solicit my support. Unspoken is: *"You're with me on this, right, doctor? You know she has to quit it with the pot. Tell her!"*

Georgina has been referred to me by a walk-in clinic for psychiatric follow-up for "depression and suicidal thoughts." She has also been referred to counseling and has been placed on Antidepressants. In the referral I've learned she has been charged with misdemeanor consumption of alcohol twice in the last two months.

Before her mother shifts the conversation to her grades, Georgina herself tells me she intentionally over-dosed a year ago. There were no complications, and she has not attempted suicide since. "What's the point?" she concludes, asking no one in particular.

In other words, she is failing at everything, including suicide.

Through questioning, I have learned she has a driver's license and a part-time job. She gets along with her supervisor and coworkers. She has a brother she seems close to and has the support of both peers and teachers at school. Although she is clearly "depressed," more striking is the hopelessness she radiates. But I am not much concerned about another suicide attempt because, despite her withdrawn demeanor in this setting, she clearly has a support network.

Deciding it wouldn't be helpful to get sucked into the parent–young adult power struggle playing out before me, I ignore the mother's invitation to either join in or refute her assessment. Instead I decide to match the daughter's disengaged style. I discourse on how the paralysis of severe and prolonged hopelessness could appear disguised as "depression." I suggest it is too soon to evaluate the effects of the Antidepressants she's been taking, and recommend that she continue with them because of their stress-reducing potential. And I strongly endorse that she continue counseling. She tersely agrees to all of it.

Mother and daughter appear together again at follow-up. Georgina is the same—impassive, undemonstrative,

minimizing or denying problems. How are things going?
Fine. Any problems? No.

"How about the Antidepressants? Have you noticed
any change?"

"No."

"I actually think she's somewhat better, doctor," the
mother disagrees. "More interactive than before."

I take charge, deliberately ignoring the mother and
focusing my attention exclusively on Georgina. I drone
on about abandonment issues, hopelessness, and the
importance of therapy. Then I spring a pointed question.

"Do you ever feel like your mother doesn't want you
to grow up?"

"Yes!" Georgina instantly agrees.

Interestingly, the mother doesn't even blink. I get
the impression she's simply waiting for her girl to finish
so she can get back to expressing her own judgments.

"Here is a suggestion, Georgina," I say. "Instead of
simply sitting there and enduring your mother's lectures,
I think you need to learn how to signal that she has done
her parental duty. That she is a good enough mother."

One of the wisdoms of Dr. MacKinnon, a looming instruc-
tor from my residency days comes to mind here: "No valid
interpretation ever goes unheard." *What did he mean?*
I asked myself then, and again fifty years later. I guess
by "valid" he meant "true" and there was truth in my
observation, based as it was on my careful assessment
of her and her mother, their power struggle, and my

refusal to take sides. I instead acknowledged Georgina's maturity, her awareness of herself and her mother, and that she had the power to assuage her mother's anxiety by simply, perhaps repetitively, signaling that she was a good mom and that their relationship would endure. In effect, I was telling Georgina that she was a grown-up, no longer a kid ... which she recognized as true, as valid. She was ready to hear. And eventually Mom was as well.

Over the next year there are five more follow-up visits. Then the next summer Georgina returns to have the Antidepressant renewed. In the waiting room, I notice two striking changes: She gives me a bright, welcoming smile. And she is accompanied by her stepfather, not her mother.

Her stepfather remains in the waiting room. As the session starts she returns to her taciturn, undemonstrative ways, waiting for questions. I check in on school, job, use of substances. Her answers are terse. Then I switch to questions of a more emotional valence.

"How are things with your mother?"

"We're getting along better."

Then the critical question. "Is your mom starting to let go?"

"Yes," Georgina tells me.

I renew her prescription and remind her to reschedule in four months.

Twelve years later, she has yet to return.

Recognizing the Signs in Georgina

There are a two points to highlight here:

Trapped by Dependence

In this case it was the parent, not the child, who could not let go. Georgina was keenly aware that behind her mother's urging her to grow up were intense feelings of abandonment that she would experience as a kind of death were Georgina to become a responsible adult. Feeling trapped by her mother's dependence—hopeless and helpless—she began to think of suicide. Her failure at that led to further feelings of helplessness. Finally she arrived at the "solution" of drugs and alcohol to help distance her from her mother's unexpressed but powerful pleas for Georgina to forever remain a child in need of constant mothering.

Coping with Mixed Messages

Even under ordinary circumstances, graduation from high school is a time of ambivalence for both parent and student, a mixture of joy and dread. *Now what?* both parties feel and think. For perhaps the first time, their relationship encounters an unquestionable point of no return, no going back to the old way of adult leading, child following. Now there is a new way: adult negotiating with adult. If the relationship is buttressed by a reasonable degree of trust—a "good enough" relationship in Winnicott's[3] terminology—parent and student will bridge the transition more or less smoothly.

But there was a trust deficiency in Georgina's world, a world dominated by her mother's entangling, dependent personality that left little room for Georgina to mature. Perhaps it would be more accurate to state that the mother's personality prevented her from recognizing her child's maturation; that is, the fact that she had found work and was getting along well with her teachers and coworkers.

Thus as graduation approached, Georgina, perceiving the transition as an abyss rather than a bridge, began to flounder. Her use of alcohol and marijuana did not protect her from freezing up under the stress of her mother's mixed message: *I expect you to succeed—although it will kill me.*

Fortunately, Georgina's capacity to trust was not completely obliterated. She was able to accept the support provided by her counselor, her work, and a boyfriend, and she navigated the gulf without crashing. And her mother was ultimately able to let go.

---

3. See *Attachment Disability Volume 1,* pp. 7–9.

Your Takeaways

With entanglement, others' needs dominate your needs.

▲

The empathy of Attachment Entanglement can paralyze, even destroy people.

▲

Cutting is always a sign of Attachment Entanglement.

▲

A social support vacuum breeds suicide potential.

▲

"Good enough" parenting does not require perfection for the child's survival, only adequacy. The same is true of therapists.

▲

Stagecraft requires modulating the degree of intimacy versus distance from the individual in order to retain their attention.

3

Attachment Disability #3:

Attachment Acting-Out

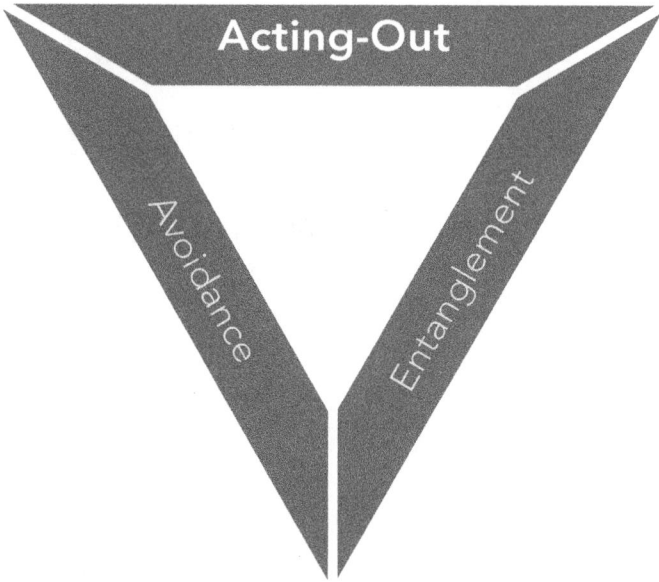

Acting-Out

Avoidance

Entanglement

Attachment Acting-Out Defined

*This type of Attachment Disability brings in ele*ments of the other two corners of the triad, Entanglement and Avoidance. What makes Acting-Out Attachment Disability unique is its basic dynamic of ambivalence. People who are affected by this variety are deeply attached, but ambivalently so.

Ambivalence is simultaneous attraction to and repulsion from an object, person, or action. It results from longing to attach but being terrified by the impulse to do so. The solution to this dilemma becomes establishing a perimeter of angry behavior and rebellious manipulation. Fear of recurrent loss becomes cloaked in anger. In contrast to the avoidant and entangled forms of Attachment Disability, where any powerful emotion—such as fear, guilt, sadness, joy, desire, or love—is threatening, here anger is safe.

This disruptiveness—often labeled "oppositional" by professionals—is a disguised plea for help and support.

Disrespectful and defiant behavior serves a second function as well; it is a manipulative, indirect way to ask for love. When it comes to children experiencing this form of Attachment Disability, an acting-out child has no less need for perceptive attentiveness than anyone else. When those in the role of parent, guardian, or any other figure assuming responsibility for supporting the child respond angrily in kind, they can later become flooded with guilt; they apologize and try to make up, displaying their love and caring on their sleeve.

The good news about this point on the triad is that Acting-Out Attachment Disability has a much better prognosis than the other varieties. Although these individuals may engage in risky behavior, they are less likely to progress to self-mutilating or suicidal behavior.

In fact, many adults with this background, assuming they have survived young adulthood without some sort of irremediable disaster—a felony record, say, or a disabling injury—evolve into law-and-order pillars of the community: police officers, attorneys, probation officers, and the like.

Case Study: Lara

"I seem to be less angry since I started taking the pills," Lara tells me. "And I have fewer headaches, so that's good."

"You are less touchy lately," Lara's mother acknowledges. "It took a few months, but I think it's helping now."

Lara is a thirteen-year-old referred to me for follow-up on Antidepressant therapy begun by another psychiatrist several months earlier.

I've received Lara's history in the referral. The headaches were the first sign of trouble. Then she started cutting. (As I noted in the previous chapter, cutting is always a sign of entanglement, and here we have another example showing that Attachment Disability is most often a blend of two or more of the three types.) Then, abruptly—and very uncharacteristically—she started talking back to her mother.

Next it was yelling and throwing things when she didn't get her way at home or didn't like what her mother was saying to her. This behavior moved into the school setting, where she started talking back to teachers and disrupting classes. Then Lara started drinking, and when her mother confronted her about it, Lara screamed at her and threatened that if she didn't leave her alone she was going to run away. Similar confrontations followed. This alarming escalation from headaches to drinking and screaming arguments had taken place over the course of just three months.

Lara's mother is a perceptive parent who has herself been in therapy off and on throughout her adult life. After we discuss the apparent success of Lara's medication regimen, her mother turns to me.

"I don't know if this information was in the referral you received, but I think it's important for you to have this background. I kept racking my brain trying to figure out how all this started, what could have happened to trigger these changes in Lara. I've been mulling over the time frame and trying to remember what else was going on then. It finally dawned on me that there was something in particular, and I checked it out with Lara. She thinks I could be right." She looked at her daughter. "Lara, do you want to tell him? I could do it, but maybe it would be good for the doctor to hear it in your own words."

"Okay," Lara agrees.

I can't help but notice that the two seem supportive of one another. It bodes well for healing Lara's trust issues.

Lara turns her attention to me. "Okay, so, my dad is one of these guys who likes to do extreme sports. You know, the kinds of things that are really out there and most people would never do them in their entire life. Like mountain boarding—do you know what that is?" she asks.

I admit I don't know.

"It's skateboarding *on a mountain*," she says, piercing me with a wide-eyed stare. "Like, skateboard racing, only *down a mountainside*. How insane is that?"

It's plain the question is rhetorical, so instead of answering it I repeat it. "So that seems crazy to you."

"Well yeah, I mean, you could break your neck. *Easy.*

So what my mom's talking about, what she figured out, is that when I first started having headaches and ... acting weird ... it was when he went on a long trip in the mountains. He told me he was going to do climbing and mountain boarding. And he was going to be gone for a really long time."

"And you worried about him," I say.

Lara nods.

"She took it pretty hard," Lara's mother offers. "But it wasn't the first time he'd done risky things. He'd gone off parasailing before, and scuba diving—"

"But he'd never left us like that for so long before," Lara interrupts. "And we had no way to reach him up there in the ... wherever he was. Yeah, it worried me. It scared me."

She finished the tale with a fair amount of heat. "And it pissed me off!"

Recognizing the Signs in Lara

Secure attachments promote trust and strengthen stress resistance, both of which are undermined when attachments are weakened. Lara clearly had a powerful reaction to her father's junket—there seems to have been more here than just the temporary loss of a supportive relationship. She apparently also experienced it as a sign of immaturity and impulsivity; hence her judgment that her father had gone "insane." As much as adolescents might decry the burdens of adult supervision—those who act out being particularly vocal about this—they expect adults to act like grown-ups. A little adult goofing around is one thing. But for Lara, doing something that could get him killed posed the threat of permanent separation.

When Lara progressed from experiencing headaches to cutting, she was substituting an external, localized discomfort for internal, diffuse but intolerable misery. When her behavior kept people at a distance, closeness was less likely—acting-out became a means of avoidance. As Helen so ably put it in the chapter on avoidance, "I've learned to keep my distance. Nobody can abandon you if you're not that close to them in the first place, right?"

Fortunately, Lara's perceptive and doggedly support-ive mother was able to read her behavioral subtext and uncover the underlying distress. No doubt the Antidepres-sant helped as well by reducing the stress and anxiety associated with the possibility of loss. With these two arrows in her quiver, Lara was able to negotiate supportive bonding without sacrificing her independence, a com-promise solution between avoidance and entanglement.

Case Study: Rita

Rita has been referred to me by her therapist, who told me she is concerned about Rita's "crazy behavior." Perhaps medication can help settle her down enough, the therapist suggests, that they will be able to make some progress in therapy. So far it's just been a lot of constructive-sounding talk but with no actual relief or change in behavior.

Rita arrives with her two-year-old daughter. She settles

the girl in the small, colorful play area in my office. I gesture toward the chair across from mine and invite Rita to sit down. She is well dressed and well groomed, forthright, and spontaneous. An obviously intelligent, thoughtful woman, she is attentive to her young child, who is very well behaved, immediately busy playing with toys.

Rita's demeanor and her interview behavior stand in marked contrast to the unsettling history I have received, sketchy though it is. I ask her to provide a more complete picture.

"Let's start by talking about what's going on with you now, your recent history."

"Okay," Rita says without hesitation. "What do you want to know?"

"Let's start with what made you decide to pursue therapy."

"There were a lot of things—I should say there *are* a lot of things. Mainly, I have a real angry streak. So many things can set me off. I try to tamp it down, but then it builds up inside anyway and I just blow up. Without warning, I may add. I don't even know it's coming myself until it's out there.

"Anger isn't all of it though. I'm afraid a lot of the time too, anxious, on edge. Other times I just feel so, so depressed. I don't even want to get out of bed."

"That's a lot to cope with," I suggest.

"Yeah, I have the works going on, don't I? I'm a regular buffet of neuroses." She smiles at her joke but I notice tears welling up in her eyes.

"I can't *sleep* either," she continues with energy. "That makes everything harder. A lot of that is probably about money, I think. I have a hard time staying employed—I'm out of work right now, in fact. It puts a lot of strain on my partner, Joseph. He's working so many hours now to keep us afloat. I wish I could help more. But I just, I just get overwhelmed too often, and then I do crazy shit."

"What kind of crazy shit? Can you give me an example?"

"Well, on the job thing, I get irritated and then snap at people. Bosses included. That's not exactly a prescription for long-term employment."

"I would have to agree with you there," I respond. "What about outside of work?"

"Okay, so a couple weeks ago I just disappeared for twenty-four hours, left Joseph with the baby. I wound up at a biker bar at one point, had a drink—I don't drink a lot but I decided to that night—and then I picked a fight with some biker chicks hanging around outside. I mean, for no reason. I don't even remember what I said, but one of them told me she was going to kick my ass. I just said, 'Be my guest.' She was going to do it, too, but the bouncer heard the yelling and came outside and broke it up."

Deliberately provoking a fight, then. "Have you done things like that before, picking fights with people, irritating them on purpose?"

"Yeah, I do that. It's all part of the big buffet you get with me."

Again, a wry smile, no tears this time.

"I get this weird satisfaction from bugging people. I even do it with Joseph, and he's so good to me, he doesn't deserve it at all. Honestly, I don't know why he stays with me. But he does. He says he's not giving up."

"Okay, I'm starting to get a picture of how difficult life is for you right now. Let's go back in time for a minute. Have you always been this volatile?"

"Honestly, I don't remember a whole lot from my childhood but my mom says I was always a 'troubled' child—her word. I started therapy when I was a teenager, and it actually worked out okay for a while. I was taking medications then too, which also helped."

"You say it worked out for a while. When did it stop working out?"

Her expression darkens. She glances over at her daughter, who is intently trying to fit colored blocks of differing shapes into corresponding holes. She turns back toward me.

"I was babysitting for my sister. I went to check on her baby girl and found her dead."

I groan audibly. "That's awful."

"Three months old." Rita sighs deeply. "It wasn't my fault, I know that. It happens, there's a name for it: Sudden Infant Death Syndrome. But I couldn't handle it."

"How did things change after the baby died?" I probe gently.

"I dropped out of treatment. Started hanging around with people on the fringes. Slackers, dropouts, drug dealers, people like that. If I hadn't met Joseph, I'd probably still be … well, who knows where I'd be. But I met him, and we got pregnant, and I have a family now. I think it's keeping me together. To the extent that I am, that is. I do manage to keep it together a lot of the time."

Recognizing the Signs in Rita

Rita's history of the significant trauma she endured, along with her mother's hints of a "troubled" childhood, certainly suggest abandonment issues. With this hunch, I make Attachment Disability the focus of the interview. Does she have trouble trusting and accepting affection or respect? I ask. Does she push people away with her behavior? She freely admits that she uses off-putting behavior as a device to manage caring relationships, that she feels safer behind a wall of provocative and irritating stunts. Here is powerful confirmation of an emotional disability resulting from unresolved attachment conflicts.

That Rita fully recognizes her emotional problems—her "buffet" of distress and her acting-out—is a huge plus when it comes to managing her disability. She has realized some *clarification*, the first step in managing Attachment Disability, which you will learn more about in chapter 5. Next she needs to practice the second step, *acceptance*, learning that her concerns about trusting are deep seated without blaming herself for this vulnerability. She needs to avoid thinking, *Why do I have trust issues?* and instead declare, *I have trust issues!* In therapist-speak, she has to *own the pain without the blame*.

I feel confident that, given what Rita has going for her—intelligence, awareness, and support—once she has spent some time practicing self-acceptance, she can move on to the third management principle: *focus* on what she might be able to change in her life to make her disability easier to manage. I hope she will learn to negotiate boundaries with words rather than behavior.

Case Study: Maddie

"I feel blank in my head. Neutral. Like there's nothing up there," Maddie says.

Her hair is magenta today. The color varies from visit to visit, but it's always a bright, unnatural color, suggesting a resistive and rebellious spirit. But the hair belies a different adolescent girl, one who is tense, anxious, restless—I would even go so far as to say haunted. Maddie is bearing a heavy burden. Her foster father is unemployed because of health issues. Her younger foster sister is severely disabled from lupus. Maddie is a very sad girl with many worries who, in addition to everything else, is also coping with a recent trauma.

I nod in acknowledgment. "That may be an effect of the Antidepressant. How about this. Why don't you stop taking the medication and come back in two weeks' time? We'll see how you're feeling then."

I have been seeing Maddie because she is exhibiting self-destructive behavior: cutting and taking drugs. Her schoolwork has taken a steep dive as well. She is seeing a therapist, and the therapist has suggested medication could offer further support. That's how I've entered the picture.

During the next session, Maddie has less of that "blank" feeling, but her anxiety level is high. Having learned from her therapist of a precipitating event to her downward spin, and suspecting Attachment Disability, I gently probe Maddie about it. Though she is clearly reluctant, I manage to extract the broad strokes of the story. She had been at a swimming hole with a gang of schoolmate friends, some of whom were diving off a cliff into the river. One boy hit his head on a rock on his way into the water, was knocked unconscious, and drowned. No one had seen it happen, so no one attempted a rescue. But everyone, including Maddie, was there when they found his body. They were all shocked, of course, but for Maddie, the event triggered a persistent withdrawal and, evidently, also precipitated the cutting, drugs, and trouble keeping up at school.

"I have memories," she concludes after telling me what happened. "They're terrible. I keep seeing pictures in my mind over and over, especially these other two boys dragging him out, and he looked so … I don't want to see that anymore, but my mind is always running. And once I start thinking about the accident, I wind up thinking about other bad things, things that happened a long time ago … when I was younger."

"What kinds of things?"

"I don't want to talk about that," she says immediately, seeming to regret having brought it up. "In fact, I don't want to talk about any of this anymore. I'm done." She folds her arms across her slumped chest.

I decide to let it go. "Maybe you can talk with your therapist about it the next time you see her."

"I don't want to do that either. She'll try to fix it. She always wants to fix things—and you can't fix stuff that already happened. Besides … it'll freak her out."

I ignore the last statement, a sign of entangling with the feelings of others, but I address her first point.

"It's true that you can't fix what's already happened," I agree. "But you can find ways to accept it and then move on. You really can. I've seen it happen again and again."

She looks at me hopefully, quiet for a moment as she turns this new idea over in her mind.

"But for right now, let's try a different medicine," I suggest, "see if it will give you a measure of relief in the near term."

I see Maddie several more times over the next few months, adjusting her prescription each time. During this period, her behavior changes dramatically and she steps up her appointments with her therapist. She has moved rapidly from withdrawal to obvious acting-out behavior, her temperament quickly ramping up to match her Day-Glo hair. She starts picking fights with her foster father and others. She threatens to do reckless things if she doesn't get her way. She storms around the house, daring anyone to cross her and reacting to imagined slights with loud, red-faced outbursts.

But Maddie, though she doesn't know it yet, is blessed. Her foster father is tolerant, insightful, and patient. He has decided to stay at her side despite her efforts to push him away, and to help her navigate this turbulent time. I will later learn what enabled him to take this approach, to remain a steadying force amid the vortex of drama: he was determined not to make the same mistakes with Maddie that he had made years earlier with a son by another relationship.

Her father's wisdom comes into play when Maddie

makes what turns out to be her last threat of this volatile period.

She arrives for her session two months after our last visit with her foster father in tow.

"You're doing a lot better, aren't you, Mads," the father says as we get started.

"Yeah, I am," she agrees. She looks at me. "Maybe we can lower my prescription again—or maybe even take me off it?"

"Sure, let's look at that," I say. "First, how about you tell me how things have been going since last time."

She takes a minute to think.

"Tell the doc what happened the other week," the father suggests. "You know, your 'sleepover.'"

Maddie snorts a laugh and looks at her father. He grins back.

"Okay, I guess I have to," she says.

Their mutual affection is evident—they strike me not as parent and child, more like a couple of old friends about to retell a favorite story.

"Okay, so, as you know, I've been doing a lot of … obnoxious things. My favorite thing has been to make threats at home. I don't think I've told you much about that."

"That's true," I say, "not much."

"Okay, so, just a couple examples … My dad told me I had to stay home and do homework while my friends were at the movies, and I told him if he didn't let me go, I was gonna chop off all my hair. That was one time. Then I told him if he wouldn't let me go hang out with my boyfriend after ten at night—and he doesn't even get off work until eight—I was gonna skip school one day and go get a tattoo." She smirks and eyes her father again. "Of *the devil!*"

Her father barks out a laugh. "Yeah, that was a good one." He turns to me. "On her forehead, she swears to me. Not a great career move."

"Well, this last time …" She pauses, considering those words. "And I guess it really was the last time, wasn't it Dad? Wow, and that was a while ago, like three weeks or something. Anyway, this time I tell him if he doesn't let me spend the whole weekend with my boyfriend, I'm going to run away with him. He has a motorcycle, and I tell my dad we'll drive off on his bike and he'll never see me again." She looks at her foster father again, hesitating. Her face flushes and she falls silent.

"And what happened when you threatened to do that, to go away forever?" I prod.

"It was the last thing I expected," she resumes. He says to me, 'I don't think that's a good idea, but I'm not going to stop you.' And I'm like 'What!' And he says 'Go ahead, go.'

"So for some reason that makes me even madder, and I say 'Fine!' and I walk out the door and slam it and run down the steps. It made a really loud bang. The neighbor came out onto her porch to look."

Maddie stops and turns toward her father again. "You finish it," she says. "I can't. I mean, it's funny now, but it's *so* embarrassing."

Her dad obliges. "Twenty minutes later, she's back—

and there are two police officers with her, one in front, one behind. The first one in the door says, 'We had a call there's an abuse situation here.'"

Maddie covers her face with her hands and shakes her head.

"Aha. Maddie called them," I conclude.

"Yup, she sure did. That'll fix me, right? Get me in trouble with the police. Only I tell them what really happened, and guess which one of us they believe."

"They believed him, of course," Maddie resumes. "But I thought I could convince them. I acted all scared and I said, 'I'm telling you, I'm not safe here, he's going to hurt me, I need you to take me to another foster home—*right now!*'"

"But the police had a different idea," the father chimes in, "and I supported it wholeheartedly. They took her to detention, and they kept her there for the whole weekend. She had to sleep in a strange bed and do a lot of chores that she just hated—"

"—It was like boot camp," Maddie finishes. "Only I bet the food was worse than what the soldiers get."

That was Maddie's last visit. Later I read that she graduated with honors and has been awarded a partial scholarship.

Recognizing the Signs in Maddie

Maddie's yelling, threats, and all-around off-putting behavior is typical of the acting-out youngster: dramatic acts designed to keep others at arm's length. She and the people whom her behavior affected were all lucky that it was short lived, that she moved through the first two steps in managing Attachment Disability, clarification and acceptance, fairly quickly. This left her in a good position to tackle the third step, learning what works for her and focusing on those solutions.

It seems clear that her father giving her permission to leave—in other words, treating her like a grown-up—turned things around. It would be interesting to have her explain why, but she herself might have no awareness of how this event freed her from her traumatic paralysis, only that things are different now. I suspect that her father, recognizing he had no control over her and that he trusted her, helped her realize she had no control over the friend who chose to dive off a cliff and drowned, that she was not to blame, that life is unpredictable. Of course she would never forget what happened, but she would remember it with sadness, not be trapped by guilt.

Case Study: Ben

Ben and his grandmother sit across from me. None of us is having a good time.

"I'm not going to take that stuff," Ben says, referring to medication I had prescribed for his resistive and defiant behavior.

"Is it not making a difference? Or are you experiencing side effects?" I ask.

"It's making a difference, but I don't like it. You could call it a side effect, maybe. I've lost my anger. I agree with people too much. It's scary."

The grandmother shakes her head in disgust. "You're

mellower these days, but that's a *good* thing. Aren't you relieved that you don't have to be fighting all the time?"

Ben has been more or less abandoned by both of his parents. It's easy to imagine they found him rather hard to love, given his attitude. His grandmother has taken him in and seems determined not to give up on him, though her frustration is apparent.

The grandmother's logic seems sound. Getting along is certainly easier than fighting all the time. But Attachment Disability has its own logic. If he continues to agree with others, build trust, and develop connections, he becomes more vulnerable to the abandonment and loss that, in his experience, are inevitable. It's better, more comfortable, to remain safe behind a wall of sulky, irritating, and provocative behavior.

There are two ways I can go with this refusal to take the medication: insist on it, or accept it. The former is the more traditional way: with adolescents you set limits and stick to them. That's how you convey that you care, which, according to theory, is what they need. This is how you build trust.

The other way is game theory, as promulgated by Gregory Bateson, Jay Haley, and others. The gist of it is that if you can neutralize/defeat the patient's attempts to be sick, the only option remaining is to get well. I decide to go the gamesmanship way: it's more interesting, and besides, I'm getting too old to be a cop.

"Okay," I say, "it's not such a bad idea. Let's have you stop taking the medication, then come back in a month and let me know how things are going. This way you'll have a chance to compare how you do with it and without it."

To my mild surprise he shows up a month later, this time alone. "I want to take the pill," he says immediately after taking a seat. "things went better in school with it."

I notice he is definitely less sulky than he'd been during our last visit. In fact, he looks lonely. Eventually what comes across is an immense sadness. I rewrite the prescription, resisting the temptation to celebrate the return of the prodigal.

"All right, let's do this again. Come back in a month," I say, "and we'll see how things are going for you."

The Dangers of Improvement

What is going on here? The games model of therapy—exemplified by Bateson—suggests that as long as Ben feels powerless, not in charge, in effect "losing," he will continue to resist.[4] His resistance has been a way for him to feel empowered, in control, a way of maintaining identity. By making the choice his own, we sidestepped his need to resist—he no longer had anything to resist against. When I let him "win," in the form of making his own treatment decisions, he gains a new identity. And in the process of winning he experiences what it's like to be a free agent. This is gratifying, perhaps, but it is also lonely. It can even be terrifying.

Another way to conceptualize this is to say he simply exercised the control he already possessed, since if he is

---

4. See *Attachment Disability Volume 1*, pp. 346–47 and 388.

really against medications, no one has the power to make him take them. What has happened is that he has been allowed to *experience choice*, which offers him a crucial opportunity: the opportunity to learn.

For Ben, accepting the medication was dangerous because it symbolized depending on an external agency to obtain control; that is, it was a surrender of autonomy. When he had the option of taking control himself, he discovered he actually lost freedom because without the drug, his disabilities returned. But in that experience he learned about himself. He learned the fact—and I think this was one reason for his sadness—that the safety of freedom also meant being alone. So he returned to resume the medication that would help him tolerate the anxieties of relationships.

There is a paradox here: by exercising his choice not to be "free" and to take medications, he began to travel the path to freedom—not freedom from anxiety, but freedom bestowed by having options with which to manage anxiety and relationships, and, by extension, life's challenges and adventures.

Your Takeaways

Attachment Acting-Out is characterized by ambivalence: those affected are deeply attached but terrified by the impulse to attach.

▲

Disruptiveness is a disguised plea for help and support.

▲

Unmet needs drive "oppositional" behavior.

▲

Adolescents expect and need Mom and Dad to be grown up.

▲

Provocativeness hides abandonment fears; anger is safe.

▲

Secure attachments promote trust and strengthen self-confidence; both are undermined when attachments are weakened.

Part II

Managing Attachment Disability

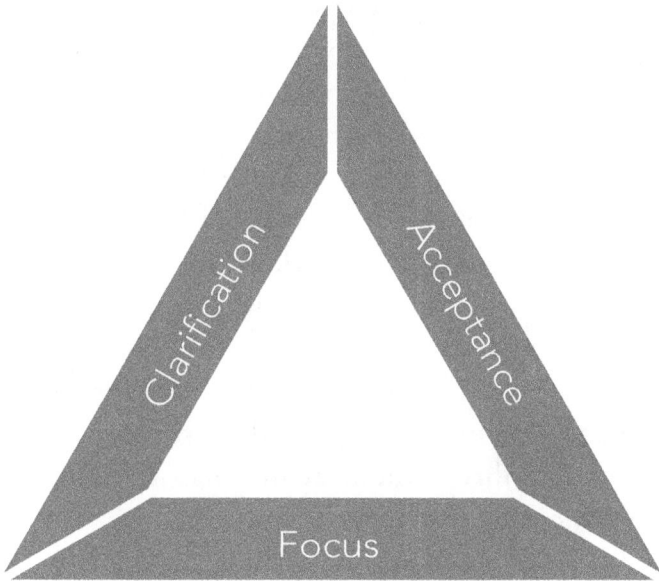

The profiles you encountered in part I are typical of those I see in people who are struggling with Attachment Disability. It is clear that the trauma that led to their difficulties in forging and maintaining healthy relationships cannot be "erased": in other words, Attachment Disability cannot be "cured." But those who are affected by it can and do learn how to live successfully with it, crowding out certain patterns of disabling behavior they developed in response to the originating trauma by balancing them with more adaptive habits. Over the long term, the key lies not in diagnosis and treatment, but in *understanding* and *managing* the disability. That is the subject of Part II, which comprises four chapters. We will start with an introductory overview of strategy and tactics. Each of the next three chapters is devoted to addressing one corner of the triad of management: *clarifying* the disability, *accepting* the disability without blame, and *focusing* on what can be changed.

Experienced therapists and counselors will immediately recognize these corners of the triad as the foundation of all effective psychotherapeutic strategies. Moreover, anyone familiar with Alcoholics Anonymous will recognize their similarity to the request for guidance expressed in the Serenity Prayer: *wisdom, serenity, courage.*

However, the majority of attachment-disabled children and adults will not have the benefit of such therapeutic expertise or guidance from a higher power. In my experience, their care, by design or default, will fall to professionals, sponsors, and family members who are unfamiliar with such concepts, and they will need management guidelines.

I will examine each of the management principles in greater detail. But it is important to first note that recovery from disability of any sort, whether physical or emotional, is quite variable because it is a function of learning, the speed of which varies from person to person. Moreover, the processes are not sequential; they loop back on each other. Recovery is not akin to retracing a circle, but to walking up a spiral where the ground is both unfamiliar yet familiar because you have gained a perspective from which to view the past and anticipate the future with some equanimity.

4

Managing Attachment Disability: Strategy and Tactics

*Whether medical or psychological, disability is usually dis-*cussed from the viewpoint of *diagnosis* and *treatment*. However, Attachment Disability does not easily fit into these categories. I recommend a different point of view, one that does not investigate the afflicted person's problems in isolation but in context. We need to see these problems in relation to the environment in which they emerged in order to conceptualize them as misfired adaptive responses. This is why I suggest we replace the paradigm of diagnosis and treatment with a more effective one: *understanding* and *management*.

Understanding

Instead of *diagnosis*, I choose this term for two reasons. First, to promote constant awareness that we are dealing with individuals whose *ability to trust is wounded* as a result of the trauma of abandonment, loss, or abuse, alone or in combination. Secondly, I choose to emphasize that trauma is the *disease*—perhaps now manifested in the form of an altered brain configuration—while impaired trust is the *disability*. Distrust is not always obvious, of course, which is why in part I, I presented a number of case studies to illustrate the many faces of wounded trust. Helping those who suffer from Attachment Disability understand the ways in which mistrust impacts their lives is a key principle of healing trust issues.

Management

I use this term to highlight the principal goal of treating Attachment Disability: *avoid making things worse.* Attachment Disability implies vulnerability. Fear of subsequent relationships is a *normal* response to any of the above unhappy life events. *It is important not to mistake disability for disease.*

Because of the vulnerability that results from trauma, subsequent offers of support may elicit wariness and concerns about being hurt again and, in extreme situations, generate distrust bordering on paranoia. Rather, the goal here is to normalize apparent pathological behavior. Paranoid distrust and hallucinations, while not uncommon, may represent a reaction to deprivation, trauma, and abuse. While such experiences may be distressing, mental health professionals should not categorize them as illness but as a variety of human experience that needs to be processed rather than treated as abnormal. Note that this does not rule out the role of medication, which some may choose in order to minimize their disability.

In other words, it is time for a different approach, time for outside-of-the-box thinking when it comes to "treatment" of the distrust that is the inevitable consequence of relationship injury. In medicine we carefully distinguish between disease and disability; for example, between an injury and its associated pain. We are taught to view the latter as a sign of tissue damage imposed by the former. Here *physical* pain signals disease, so when patients complain of pain, we doctors search for disease. However, as counselors sometimes we muddle this distinction and come to view *emotional* pain and suffering—the disability itself—as the core problem. This puts us at risk of not recognizing an underlying trauma.

The Principle at the Heart of Management

Your goal in managing Attachment Disability is this: *Avoid making things worse.*

Put another way, you must be careful to avoid reinforcing the attachment-disabled individual's maladaptive behaviors. Why is this the bottom line? Because if you can avoid doing that, behaviors that are more adaptive will spontaneously flourish, driven by the activating energies of unmet needs. Given time and effort, constructive behaviors will crowd out and displace destructive ones.

Understand Your Constraints

That sounds simple, doesn't it? But this simple plan is not easily executed. So here, my aim is to offer guidelines, based on my own successes and missteps over the years, for how to approach this task, and the place I'd like to start is with *understanding your constraints*.

To effectively manage traumatized children, adolescents, and adults, *you* need to acquire a certain set of skills that will enable you to address these constraints. You must learn to:

- Recognize their power to resist
- Deal with their inattentiveness
- Time your feedback

We'll take these one at a time.

Management Strategy: The Three Constraints

Constraint #1: The Power to Resist

Recognize the autonomy of the person in your office who presents with Attachment Disability. No matter which of the three varieties they evince, they always have the power to resist engaging with you. Human transactions do not occur by chance. Rather, they are driven—activated—by unmet needs. Transactions thus involve the exchange of needed goods and services, hopefully by agreement, which is the basis of social organization. Peaceful exchanges proceed via a reciprocal exchange of power. But each of the parties always has the power to resist.

People beset by attachment issues are prone to resist because of their distrust of power and authority. Bitter experience has taught them that transactions risk entanglement, betrayal, abuse, or abandonment, typically combining elements of each. It is simply safer to resist. *If you trust*, they have learned, *you lose.*

What this means in practice is that parents, teachers, and counselors intending to help must guard against being seduced by the power of their position. No matter the honors or responsibilities, formal or informal, that accrue to us via society's favor or laws, those nominally subordinate to us always retain the power to resist—for example, tune out, skip class, become truant, or drop out of therapy. Thus, take care to approach all interactions *without* an expectation of automatic obedience.

Constraint #2: Attentiveness

Let me provide a frame for this constraint by returning to my training years and the topic of countertransference. In our bull sessions as residents, we not infrequently addressed the issue of how to deal with attractive patients. How do you resist the seductiveness of intelligence or beauty? How do you avoid being snared by the very traits that no doubt played a part in bringing the patient to your office for help? I can't recall any of us coming up with a definitive answer. Nor did our professors. Yes, they would agree, that can be a problem, but it is something you need to discuss with your analyst to understand better what your conflicts are. Not having an analyst, I never did find out what conflict had to do with the attraction of one human being to another, although it was clear that attraction could generate conflict; hence our question.

Well, once in practice I discovered I was, indeed, very susceptible to seduction ... *by attentiveness.* I was a sucker for the patient who in the course of an interview might say something like, "Dr. Curran, I was thinking about what you said before." My pulse would accelerate, my pupils dilate, my thinking transfixed by loving surrender: *Oh, what a beautiful, perceptive being it is that worships before me.* Whether the patient agreed or disagreed with my observations was irrelevant. The listening: that was what was significant, for it offered the possibility of developing a treatment contract. Now we could proceed to explore the data upon which the patient's opinion was based. Where did we agree and why? Where did we disagree and why? Now we were both poised to learn.

On the other hand, take the situation of someone, no matter how good looking or smart, chattering on regardless of the astuteness of my prior observations. The result: I feel ignored, at risk of tuning out. As a human being I need recognition, and you need recognition too. Lack of recognition from a patient has the potential to undermine a therapeutic relationship. If you surrender to your client's inattentiveness with a corresponding lack of attention, no learning—which is the goal of disability management—will take place. You must remain vigilant and be prepared to tactfully interrupt, and restructure and refocus the proceedings. I will provide examples of restructuring interventions in chapter 5 on clarification.

Lack of attentiveness can take a variety of forms. It helps if you understand, for example, why a client might flood you with words and irrelevancies, ignoring your responses and questions. This behavior most often represents underlying abandonment issues. Such clients feel overwhelmed by a need to "get everything in" before you disappear from their life, which is their experience. Should you actually tune out—begin to mull over your plans for your evening or weekend, for example—they will sense your inattentiveness, and, now feeling abandoned, intensify their verbosity.

Someone experiencing hopelessness may communicate lack of attentiveness in a different way, by being distracted, waiting to be prompted to speak, holding back. Again, refocusing is called for.

If your attempts to refocus and restructure do not succeed in gaining the person's attention, you must consider the possibility that more than abandonment disability is present: behind the inability to focus may be intoxication from prescription drugs or other substances, developmental issues, impending psychotic decompensation, or other factors. You will need to address any such underlying cause before you can move ahead with disability management, and this might entail a consultation referral to a colleague while you continue your work.

Constraint #3: Timing

The timing with which you express the insights and suggestions that emerge in your work with an attachment-disabled person can be tricky. A mistimed comment during a session can be intrusive, as can a failure to comment at all. Conversely, an intuitive remark or companionable silence at the right moment can generate notable anxiety relief. Timing is much more of an art than a science—or perhaps more accurately, it is a craft. It is through practice that you will develop a feel for what is likely to work in a given situation.

You might say I had an opportunity to hone my craft when I worked with a fourteen-year-old client named Owen.

Case Study: Owen

On our first (and last) visit, his mother reports that Owen has been resistive since the age of two. In other words, even at his present young age, Owen has already been resisting authority for a dozen years.

"What brings you here?" I ask Owen.

No eye contact. "I dunno," he mumbles.

I wait expectantly, but instead of answering, Owen changes the subject, remarking distractedly about the poor layout of my office. The chair is uncomfortable. It's too dark.

The mother steps in. "Dr. V. says she can't work with him. Says she doesn't usually work with adolescents."

Owen giggles, his attitude defiant, mocking. He rolls his eyes, makes a few further snide comments about the physical setup. I am starting to understand why Dr. V. didn't want to work with him. He seems to have perfected an array of expressions that communicate he is immune to suggestion, let alone direction.

"He doesn't want to take his medicine," the mother says.

"I doubt if he *does* take it," I immediately assert.

"How did you know?" Owen smirks.

"Call it a good guess. It doesn't matter. At any rate, not taking your medicine isn't going to be a problem for me."

Owen makes full eye contact for the first time. "Hey," he says. "I like this doctor!"

The mother isn't quite as delighted as the son. "I don't think that's a good message for him to hear!"

I do my best to salvage the situation, explaining that since Owen has been willful since he was a toddler, telling him now to follow orders would be fruitless. Explaining that to address the fear behind noncompliance, you have to be able to take the issue off the table.

The mother is unimpressed. I suggest that I am perhaps not what she is looking for in a psychiatrist, and I waive my fee. The mother stands, stony faced, and turns on her heel. Owen follows her out the door without looking back.

I had played my hole card too soon. I should have finessed the issue of compliance. I should have turned to Owen, perhaps feigning surprise, with a bland inquiry: "Could your mother's allegation about not wanting to take medications possibly be true?"

This tactic softens resistiveness. Whether there is a response or not, the repetitive seeking of a response conveys a subtext: *you can't make me give up or get mad by ignoring me.*

This is where having the sponsor in the room can be critical. Engaging the sponsor via, say, taking a history, not only provides pertinent data but offers an opportunity to slowly engage the resistive party. With Owen, the idea would be to gradually undermine the desperate noncompliant posture that colored his view of grown-ups and authority. It would reflect the centrality of what noncompliance has come to mean for him in the first place: *to comply would be to lose his identity.*

I might justify overplaying my hand by saying that the history I had received on Owen plus his behavior made it clear to me from the start that a major issue here was developmental. This implied that effective management would depend primarily on Owen participating in a skills-training agenda. Or, to put the matter differently, medication was not the answer—at least not yet. That could come later; now he needed engagement. Therefore it was not dangerous to downplay the medication issue as I did, because other matters were more important.

But medication *was* the most important matter for the mother because it symbolized her hope that power emanating from a doctor could make her child behave at last. In short, my job was to be a cop.

Now, doctor-or-counselor-as-cop is an expectation not unfamiliar to any physician or counselor who deals with adolescents or young adults and their sponsors. It is important to neither buy into nor rebuff such an expectation but to gently explore its dimensions. Sponsors and parents typically experience a good deal of anxiety should their kids not be well mannered or studious. It is when one-on-one discussions have not helped that they turn to an outsider, hoping that lectures from an authority figure will make a difference, and sometimes they do.

For parents who struggle with their children's developmental issues, the anxiety-provoking potential of poor manners generally ranks high. Getting them to fit in at all, that's the issue, and it had been the issue with Owen since he was a toddler.

But the mother, obviously intelligent and motivated, also had an issue: She had not learned from experience. She had not figured out that one more exercise of authority, whether hers or others', was not going to be the answer.

I recognized this and, based on my four decades' experience with medication noncompliance, knew that if compliance remained the primary goal of treatment, the inevitable outcome would be persisting noncompliance. So, aiming to disqualify myself as an enforcer of medication compliance, I put my cards on the table, hoping that I could take compliance off that table. But I was trumped by the mother's exercise of her authority; she removed Owen from treatment.

The question remains: Could I have obtained the mother's cooperation by first addressing the compliance issue directly with her, rather than indirectly via Owen? Should I have stated there were some issues more important than medication? Should I have noted that medication was a symbol of power for both the mother and Owen—as it is for many youngsters and their parents—and that therefore the basic issue here was a power struggle? That we needed to focus on the two of them learning how to get along? I doubt it—the two were so entrenched.

Nonetheless, I could have been more patient.

Your Takeaways

Attachment Disability management requires replacing the paradigm of *diagnosis/treatment* with a more effective one: *understanding/ management.*

▲

Fear of subsequent relationships is a *normal* response to the traumas of abandonment, loss, or abuse. It is important to not misinterpret this relationship disability as disease.

▲

Your goal is to *avoid making things worse.*

▲

You need to acquire the skills to address the constraints inherent in this therapeutic relationship. You must learn to:
Recognize the person's autonomy,
their power to resist;
deal with their inattentiveness;
time your feedback.

5

Management Principle #1:
Clarification

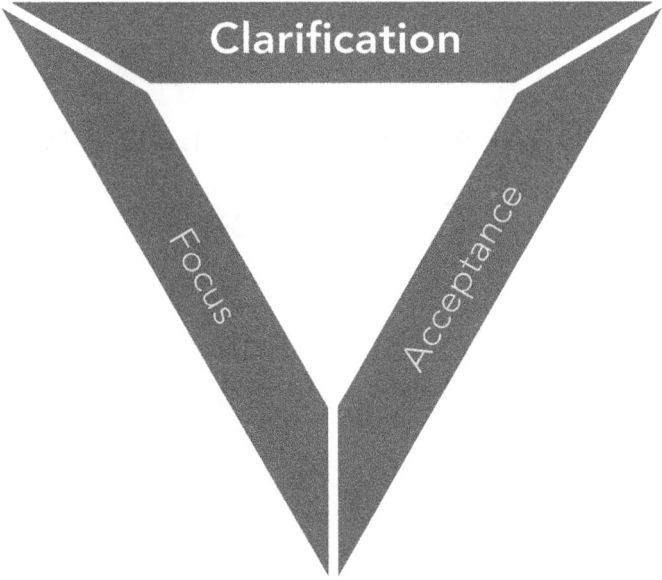

Many people are untutored when it comes to describing their suffering. They lack a vocabulary to describe their inner world and therefore resort to global words such as "unmotivated" or "procrastinating" or "upset" or "miserable" or "unhappy" or "depressed" or "stressed." While it is important to record what they have to say, you must also move beyond the general to the specifics, to the phenomena that give rise to the global complaint. This can be particularly arduous with adolescents and younger adults because they are so close to the trauma of their separation and loss. That is, the resulting anxieties not only suffocate their introspection but also make it difficult to restore the ability to attach. Instead they collapse into a state of paralysis and disability, which is what brings them to my doorstep.

What types of clarification are likely to be most helpful? These are three of the most important ones:

- Distinguishing "depression" from anxiety
- Distinguishing death preoccupation from suicidal intent
- Identifying the fears that lurk behind anger

Let's explore them in order.

Distinguishing "depression" from Anxiety

As a counselor to Attachment Disability sufferers, there are two words you will inevitably encounter when they or their parents or sponsors come to you for help: the first is "anxiety," the second "depression."

The Notion of Anxiety

Anxiety and its impact on trusting are central to this handbook. Anxiety has the power to both stimulate and suppress, to create and crush, to unite and separate. And anxiety feeds distrust.

Webster's defines anxiety as "… a painful uneasiness of mind over an impending or anticipated ill." This is a pretty handy definition; it's what I find patients generally have in mind when they use the word, although not all of them are able to connect the experience with any specific event—it seems to be "free floating" for some. It such cases it is not uncommon for anxiety to be mistaken for "depression"; some patients describe their anxiety as a "black cloud coming over me." In fact, anxiety and depression generally coexist, which I will discuss shortly.

Regardless of the language or behavior cloaking it, however, anxiety can always be understood because we all experience it. This has the advantage of drawing us together. While we truly cannot say to the other that we know *how* they feel, on the other hand we truly can say we understand *what* they feel. The idea here is to focus on the "what" of anxiety, rather than the "why" or the "how" of it. What is happening is much more important than why or how it is happening.

A Definition of Anxiety

The "what" of anxiety is this: *anxiety is always the prospect of separation.*

This dictum was conveyed to me by Dr. Lawrence Kolb, the director of the New York Psychiatric Institute (PI) during my residency training there in the 1960s, under circumstances memorable precisely because they were so mundane.[1]

---

1. Dr. Kolb was certified in medicine, neurology, psychiatry, and psychoanalysis. He served as president of the American Psychiatric Association, later as chairman of the American Board of Psychiatry and Neurology. He authored a highly respected textbook of neurology. Despite his formidable credentials, as a supervisor he radiated leadership, rather than authority, combined with a very dry sense of humor. I think he found our struggles to learn the art of therapy engaging for I always sensed a twinkle in his eyes. Not that he was reluctant to pull rank when necessary, as I found out one time when I had the temerity to ignore twice a rather pointed therapeutic suggestion. Finally he ordered, "Dr. Curran! Start lithium treatment on your patient! Look it up!" I did and the patient promptly improved enough to be discharged. It was an honor to know him and be supervised by him. (A rather charming vignette of him, which captures the essential man, is available from a former student. Druss, R. G. "Dr. Lawrence C. Kolb: One Student's Recollection." *American Journal of Psychiatry*: 2001;58 (5):692.)

   As the years passed and as I began to grasp the wisdom involved in his conception of anxiety, I was amused by the irony of receiving it not from high above on a mountaintop, but high in PI cornered in an elevator.

PI is located in a fifteen-story Art Deco tower crammed into the west end of the Columbia University medical campus, perched on a bluff overlooking the Hudson River. The tower dates from the 1920s, charming but cramped, with antiquated mechanicals. Its elevators reflected its age: pokey, inadequate, confined. One morning I was on my way to the library on a higher floor when the elevator paused and the doors opened to admit Dr. Kolb, evidently on his way to his office above.

There were just the two of us, trapped in this groaning, slowly ascending contraption. We began to chat about the different ways to conceptualize anxiety. The elevator finally reached his destination, its doors opening. He stepped out. As he turned away he tossed off a final remark: "Of course, it's all due to separation."

The elevator doors closed, and he was gone from my sight, but his words were grit in the mind's eye. Despite my respect for Dr. Kolb, I didn't buy it. I remembering thinking, *How can he be so dogmatic?* But you don't readily forget an unambiguous, authoritative declaration of this sort. I pondered the idea for a while, then filed it away, a kind of psychiatric curiosity midst the orthodoxies of that era.

Then I encountered Rebecca.

Case Study: Rebecca— Treatment-Resistive "Depression"

"I'm just so depressed," Rebecca tells me—again.

That's how she describes what she is feeling. For my part, I'm feeling gloomy and distracted. I have been listening to this complaint for a very long time. Rebecca has been seeing me off and on since 1968 when I was at Minneapolis General, treating her for phobias and depression. It's now 1982 and I'm in private practice. It is February, and as I stare out the window, I notice my mood is echoed by sinking, steel-gray clouds, threatening more snow.

Rebecca had improved for a time when I first started treating her—until her husband left her for another woman. For years thereafter, her symptoms waxed and waned. Sometimes she was paralyzed by her phobias, afraid to leave the house; at other times, she could function fairly normally. Try as I might to manage her medication, nothing I prescribed seemed to offer any lasting benefit.

Things worsened in 1975 when her father died and her sister moved in with Rebecca and her son, Marc. Her sister and Marc locked horns immediately, and Rebecca allowed herself to get sucked into their conflict. And that wasn't all: her sister constantly criticized Rebecca's parenting. In response to this one-two punch, Rebecca lived with persistent guilt, blaming herself for her inability to keep the two of them happy and questioning her worth as a parent. Her isolating phobias intensified.

She was now seven years into this seemingly impossible dynamic.

"Things are difficult at home again, I take it."

"Yes. It just never stops. I can't catch a break. I know you know that—it's not the first time you've heard it. The two of them are constantly sniping at each other. And her criticism of me as mother never lets up. Lately, she's been telling me that if I don't do something, Marc is going to turn out just like his father. I wish I could just shake it off, but I *hate* hearing that. She might be right, and it makes me feel so ... defeated."

There is no flash of lightning, no heavenly voice, yet it dawns on me that what Rebecca is reporting to me is not depression at all: it's *worry*. She's concerned that her sister could be right, that there may be nothing she can do to avert that fate for her son. And perhaps just as worrisome, that everyone will think it's *her fault*.

"Let's try something," I venture. "Why don't you use the word 'worried' instead of 'depressed'? That's what I think you're actually telling me. You're worried your sister might be right about where Marc is headed. But guess what—in reality, you have very little control over his life. The best you can do is to tell him what you think is right for him, regardless of what your sister thinks. Marc is nearly grown now. What happens after that is his responsibility."

The clarification proves to be huge. Over the next few sessions she comes to understand that much of her "depression" is actually her frustration with the older sister's second-guessing of her parenting—which happens to be a replay of criticism she received in childhood. She realizes that this hasn't made her depressed at all: it's made her *furious*. But she has been stuffing her anger, for fear of losing control and raging at her sister. She has lost her husband and she is losing her son. She cannot risk jeopardizing her only remaining attachment, as painful as it is.

In a later session, I set further rules for describing her feelings.

"I often hear you apologizing for your problems—'I should just shake it off' is one I hear a lot. And that word 'should' appears frequently when you describe your situation. I suggest you pay attention to that word and try not using it. Instead try using the word 'need' and see if that helps to sort things out."

This proves to be a very helpful clarification. Subsequently, Rebecca's fears and anxieties slowly begin to recede as she realizes they are actually understandable in the context of her life experiences. She begins to accept that it's impossible to make everyone happy. We also examine her hidden belief that her anger will be lethal if she reveals it openly, a consequence of being raised by an emotionally abusive mother.

Her improvement continues, marked by a particular milestone: one day her sister calls me to complain that Rebecca is becoming more withdrawn, not "happy." What is really going on is that Rebecca is pretending less and stuffing less and being more honest about her own conflicts and frustrations—and her anger.

Not long after, I notice with great satisfaction that Rebecca has become more direct with me and more accepting that further medication isn't going to help. The change is dramatic: she stops asking for any new cocktails to treat her "depression." In fact, that word disappears from her vocabulary. She focuses less on parenting and more on how to manage living with her unhappy and judgmental sister. She frowns and expresses frustration less often, and is even able to laugh and kid herself about how unrealistic some of her fears have been.

In short, after many years of being stalled in "depression," Rebecca is finally—and rapidly—learning how to manage her disability.

In 1985 she announced she was flying to Texas for Mark's graduation from boot camp: pretty remarkable, I thought, for a woman previously a social cripple. I have had no word of or from her since.

Learning from Rebecca

My experiences with Rebecca offer several lessons.

Never Accept an Individual's Self-Report Uncritically

Of course, you do want to record their statements in their own words. On occasion I will include extended quotes if the report is vague or unfocused or rambling, this to provide context and ambience for a later reader. At the same time, you remain alert for the underlying phenomena and life experiences that are generating the speech. If these do not appear, you might attempt a *clarifying* inquiry, perhaps preceded with a preamble, something like "You know I've been wondering what your 'depression' is like. Could you give me more details about it?" Or something like "Do you have any worries that get you down?"

Be Careful with the Timing of Your Clarifying Questions

Understand that a request for clarification (also known as reframing) can be experienced as intrusive and rejecting, as if you are not listening. Therefore, timing is important. I could be direct with Rebecca because I had worked with her for many years and had earned her trust. So she had no difficulty considering what I had in mind as soon as I offered her an alternative way to describe her experiences. But this is not always the case, of course. Sometimes a clarifying interpretation is better introduced as a somewhat offhand aside; for example, "You know sometimes when people talk about 'depression' they actually are referring to things like worries or anxieties ..." You pause for a beat or two, then go on with the dialogue. Even if there is no immediate response, your remark has not gone unheard; as one of my professors used to say, you are speaking to the unconscious because no valid interpretation goes unheard. This is so because counseling can be likened to a search for the truth in the person's life, a quest. In this sense you are a detective carrying on an investigation, not of a crime but of a functional disability. As you investigate and compile information, certain items might impress you as significant that you will eventually present to the person in a (hopefully) orderly and meaningful way. But you do not proclaim in doing so that your presentation is the "truth" of his or her life. Instead you wonder whether your assessment provides *clarification*. And then you observe.

What do you observe for? Three things. Most important, you look for distortions of your message: Does the individual seem to feel he or she is being blamed for the functional disability? If so, you restate your message, perhaps cloaked in different terminology, hoping to minimize the distortion. This may take only a minute or two, but it can sometimes take weeks or months if the disability is trauma related. This is because trauma victims are typically blamed for what befell them, or they blame themselves for it. It is ingrained, and for them a (sometimes *the*) significant "truth" of their life.

You also listen for what part of the message seems to "fit," and if so, how and why. And you listen for the parts that do not seem to fit—again, how and why. Using this feedback and the additional relevant data accompanying it, you construct an alternative scenario to present with the hope of providing further clarification, as well as *acceptance* of the trauma or disability without blame but with an increased ability to *focus* on what can be changed (the subjects of the next two chapters). In this way, as I sometimes say to my patients, "My job is to help you better understand yourself, to teach you how to be your own detective midst the mystery of your life, and to establish a life path to travel." You'll find that once people understand the grip of their attachment issues, they will develop their own explanation for why they are gripped.

Thirty-seven years have passed since my Rebecca epiphany. With certainty, I can now say that no one who has crossed my doorway since is without "worries" and anxieties. The same is true of your doorway. And for the great majority, these anxieties are more or less paralyzing, which is why they seek help to begin with. Some people will deny and minimize, but that is another issue. Every therapist and counselor has a Rebecca or two or more bogged down and ensnared by paralyzing anxiety mislabeled as "depression."

Paralyzing Anxiety Is Often Accompanied by Shame and Blame

These may be expressed in thoughts such as *What's the matter with me? Why can't I be like everyone else? Why don't I have more faith in God? Why don't I do the things I know I have to do? Why can't I be happy?* "Should" thinking is also prominent, sometimes openly expressed: "I shouldn't feel this way. I should be more active. I shouldn't feel upset." This is sustained by the person's conditioned expectation of criticism. By blaming themselves, they hope to obtain mercy; by blaming others, to escape condemnation.

Either mode is paralyzing because it shifts the power to change behavior into the hands of outsiders. Moreover, it reinforces the view of the world as a moral place; that is, one where every problem is someone's fault.

Here a second type of clarification is called for. You need to teach individuals how to be *descriptive rather than judgmental* as they review their suffering, their performance, the attitude of their family and coworkers, or whatever else they may be describing to you. Like the clarifying questions cited earlier, this can be experienced as intrusive, as well as disrespectful. Therefore, it is important to move slowly and build trust, even providing an overview of what the two of you are trying to accomplish. *Own your thoughts and feelings and behavior!* is the mantra here.

I might begin this step by modeling how to be assertive and forthright in their statements; for example, not to apologize by tone of voice or gesture as they report their experiences.

As a psychiatrist I encounter this frequently when prescribing a medication. I expect the odds are two in five that upon their return patients will report the medication did not work or had to be discontinued because of side effects; that is, they will describe what seems to be a therapeutic failure. And it is even much more likely their report will include an apology, either via word or behavior—an averted gaze or confessional tone of voice or slumping of posture—that signals guilt and self-blame. But here an apparent treatment failure provides an opportunity to practice therapeutic alchemy. That is, such behavior offers an opening to practice clarification, to undermine a self-destructive attitude that typically infects the attachment-disabled person's entire world: accepting blame for things over which they have no control.

For example, consider Maya, an exemplar of an individual who habitually apologizes whenever things do not work out as expected. In our previous meetings I have noticed and perhaps commented on this very habitual but unrealistic world view. Now she's back, troubled by a lack of benefit after trying another medication.

Case Study: Maya—
Everything Is My Fault

"It's not working," Maya tells me, looking hangdog, her tone subdued.

"Hold it," I respond, seizing the opportunity. "There you go again, apologizing."

Maya looks puzzled. Evidently, she has forgotten our previous discussions. "What?"

"Why are you apologizing? You tried the pill. You can't control how it works."

"I'm not apologizing," she says. A little irritation has bubbled up into her voice.

"Yes you are! Look at your tone of voice, how you are sitting."

She still looks confused, so I decide to show her what I'm after.

"Okay, here. Look straight at me and repeat, only louder, 'It's not working.'"

"The pill is not working," she says. There is still no energy behind the statement.

"Louder!"

"It's no good," she tries, now timidly assertive.

I point out the window at a ridge across the freeway. "Pretend I'm standing way over there and you have to shout to make me hear."

Maya struggles with this—she is embarrassed, but she gives it a try: "*No good.*"

"Again."

She is now distinctly annoyed with my persistence,

and blurts out, perhaps a bit sarcastically: "*Nooooo goood!!*"

"Very good," I say. "The reason I pushed you on this is that I wanted to show you that you have the habit of accepting fault for things you have no power to control."

Maya looks skeptical, but nods her head.

As a counselor, teacher, or other support person, you will encounter similar behavior when you have "prescribed," suggested, or recommended a therapeutic option—say meditation or imaging or perhaps consultation for a trial of medication—to your clients. Some will return to report no benefit despite good effort, signaling fault. It is most important to recognize the effort but not the implicit apology. Although this rudimentary behavior modification technique seems rather trivial, if used selectively it can have powerful effects with "depressed" individuals. Sometimes I supplement it by giving them a prescription to post on their bathroom mirror, such as: "*Describe your life, don't judge it.*" This serves as a daily reminder of the mental state they need to develop. With others, I designate a gesture I might use to prompt them to reframe an apologetic behavior or statement. I explain, "You are pretty good at judging the goodness and badness of your thoughts and feelings. Now let's see if you can develop another habit: simply describing them to yourself, 'owning' them without labeling them."

If there is a concerned partner or sponsor or parent in the person's life, I might suggest they attend the next visit to have me demonstrate the technique. Frequently such supportive parties have become somewhat demoralized themselves. They have long had to cope with their loved one's negative talk and demeanor, and with their unresponsiveness to encouragement and expressions of caring. Being so rebuffed and discouraged, it is inevitable that despite the sponsor's or parent's best wishes to be supportive, irritable and impatient feelings well up, and it takes energy to control them, a fatiguing process and a prelude to burnout. Having the technique of simply describing thoughts and feelings to fall back on not only protects the sponsor but reinforces what is happening in treatment. In effect, the people who are most involved in the patients' lives become co-therapists.

This approach has its limitations, however. It works best if applied intermittently; otherwise both you and your client risk becoming fatigued. Older people might find both my behavior and the ownership I advocate too threatening—if they are not prepared. Again, timing is critical. And a few are simply afraid of raising their voice; they fear they might lose control or others will go out of control. They understand the rationale of the tactic, but to emit assertive vocalizations is threatening. And any hint of energy in their own voice recreates past abuse experiences. So they freeze up.

For others, their blaming may be so deeply entrenched and wired in that they may not be conscious of it. To address the blaming directly by describing the thought or feeling not only sails right over their head, but risks aggravating the problem: here is yet another situation that, as they appraise it, is their fault. Such people are so bogged down by anxiety that they will simply find this technique incomprehensible. In fact, it will feel like more punishment because their world is always one of fault and retaliation. This requires different management techniques, perhaps role playing. The goal is to promote the idea of a world that is not always a jungle, not always cruel or exploitative, but rather, a world in which lost souls are sometimes rescued.

For others, sometimes I suggest they replace the word *should* with the word *need*, as I suggested to Rebecca. That is, not *What should I do or think?* But rather *What do I need to do or think?* Not *How should I feel?* but *What do I need to feel?* Here the idea is to send a message that problem solving is a survival issue, not a moral one.

Childhood Abuse and Adult Disability

Nowadays everyone, professional and nonprofessional alike, is aware of the devastation of child abuse. Multiple media accounts are a daily occurrence. But forty years ago, the role of abuse in the genesis of adult psychological disability went unrecognized by psychiatry. Fortunately things have changed since then ... somewhat. Although inquiries about abuse are now a routine part of all medical and psychological evaluations, too often the emphasis is on current relationships; for example, between spouses or partners or lovers. But the residuals of childhood and adolescent abuse, whether witnessed or sustained, can later manifest in the form of serious and persisting adult disability, one aspect of which is the abused person's paradoxical clinging to the abuser.

Another complication is misdiagnosis. In Rebecca's

case the misdiagnosis was my accepting her complaint of "depression" as a textbook case of Depression. I am sure she appreciated my interest and energy, most likely the reason for her faithful compliance over the years. But she needed more.

Ultimately it became clear the emotional abuse Rebecca sustained during her childhood and adolescence paralyzed her, sucking the vitality out of her, rendering her colorless and subservient and clinging. Perhaps this is why her husband left her once she improved, figuring that now she could manage without him. But when her older, domineering sister moved in—who forecast doom regardless of circumstance and who tolerated no voice other than her own—Rebecca sustained a relapse. Once again, she was trapped

Two things can happen to youngsters raised with an abusive parent: they emulate the abuse, or they suppress it. Sometimes they do both. Emulation serves to promote distance and maintain safe boundaries, while serving as a disguised call on the environment for help. Suppression, the much more likely outcome in my experience, is actually more disabling because, as the repressed affect begins to percolate into awareness, it prompts fears of retaliation or ridicule, even obliteration should anyone—*anyone!*—suspect its presence. Any powerful emotion or feeling state—joy or satisfaction or sadness or anger or happiness—becomes threatening. In Rebecca's case, the result is colorlessness, homeboundedness, and hidden social anxiety.

Dr. Kolb's Dictum Modified

In view of the epiphany I experienced during my encounters with Rebecca and Maya and many others, I will paraphrase Dr. Kolb's pronouncement, not as a rigid law but as a rule of thumb to assist in understanding and managing emotional disability. The idea here is to get into the habit of looking beyond the behavior the person exhibits and determining whether it stems from loss and separation.

> *We can understand anxiety as the response to the prospect of change, whether immediate or pending, whether real or symbolic.*

Change always incorporates some kind of separation and loss. Think about it: not of the obvious changes that bedevil life—birth, death, marriage, relocation, school, promotion, retirement, layoff—but the very minor fluctuations we all experience in the day's flow of events: traffic jams, the headlines, our partner's behavior, the coworker who butts in, the colleague who doesn't acknowledge a friendly greeting, and so on. Each blip, or the absence of an expected blip, ignites a passing appraisal of its significance, the gist of which is this: *Does this affect the security of my relationships?* Of course, most such appraisals do not rise to the level of consciousness, unless the blips multiply and evolve into a major disruption of life's flow. Then they might ignite what I call a *What if?* thought. (A friend calls it *awfulizing*.)

The consequences of *what-iffness* thinking depends on

the context of the appraisal, factors such as our history of loss and separation, the trauma embedded in our neurons, the degree to which blame—*whose fault is it?*—rules our life, the degree of support in our environment, and so on. We might judge the blips as no threat to our security status at all. Certain blips might even motivate us to an enhanced state of performance. In short, some anxieties possess survival value.

On the other hand, we might find that certain blips signal ominous portent: the prospect of abandonment. This has the potential to trigger a body/brain combat mode that prepares us to contest the loss of security, or replace what might be lost, or both. That type of blip transforms us into a pumped-up, activated state, a state of *stress*, the duration of which can range from a few seconds to an entire lifetime. The longer the duration of this state, the more prone we are to disability. And conversely, successfully overcoming the challenges evoked by change can enhance our self-acceptance and self-confidence.

The Notion of Depression

One cornerstone of this book is injured trust. The other is the self-blaming that grips trauma survivors. The anxiety of distrust is an *emotional* process that paralyzes and degrades *one's ability to adapt*, while undermining learning. In contrast, self-blaming is a *cognitive* phenomenon, an error of judgment generated to cope with the paralysis: *It's all my fault that I am not able to ...* Of course the effort to adapt is doomed to fail, which leads to lower self-esteem, more anxiety about rejection, and more paralysis. This unhappy dynamism is frequently characterized by survivors as "depression." Most survivors do not understand or tend to minimize the paralysis.

Unfortunately, this erroneous self-assessment is too often accepted uncritically by psychiatrists and counselors as Depression, which may result in a second error of judgment: over-treatment with Antidepressants. This places survivors at risk of being shuffled down a blind alley leading to their being designated as "treatment resistant." In fact they are actually *medication resistant* since a number of effective non-pharmacological therapeutic options are available for treatment of Depression; for example, Cognitive Behavioral Therapy (CBT).

Therefore, any discussion of Attachment Disability is incomplete without some consideration of the notion of "depression."

This is a term that escapes terse characterization, reflected in *Webster*, where in contrast to anxiety, the definition of Depression is broader: "... dejection, as of mind ... lowering of vitality or functional activity ... negative attitude ... abnormal state of inactivity and unpleasant emotion ..." Interestingly, as unwieldy as it is, the definition accurately reflects the dual nature of Depression, involving both psychological and physical impacts.

In fact, everyday use of the term is even broader than *Webster*. Attachment-disabled youngsters and adults also make use of it as they refer to stress and anxiety phenomena such as minute-to-minute changes in feelings, worry, looming apprehension, and so on. Indeed, surveys suggest that 48 to 78 percent of Depressive illness is accompanied by an anxiety disorder. But not infrequently, individuals cram all issues of whatever sort into the portmanteau of "depression." This is what derailed my treatment of Rebecca for years: my acceptance at face value of her use of the word "depression" to denote her suffering.

Yet it is really impossible to carry on a discussion with an attachment-disabled person or those supporting them—or to author a handbook, for that matter—without using the term. Hence, when I enclose the term *in quotes*, I refer to its *popular commonplace use* in everyday conversation. But when I use the term *capitalized without quotation marks*, I have in mind its more *technical meaning* within the professions.[2]

- Popular use = some kind of uncomfortable feeling or behavior, accompanied by some degree of functional paralysis, signified by quotes: "depression."
- Technical use = as defined in standard psychiatric textbooks, useful for academic and administrative purposes, signified by uppercase: Depression

(Confusing? Of course, but this is what happens when we confuse words with the reality they are intended to signify. This is what the ancient Greeks had in mind when they said you could not step into the same river twice.)

Accordingly, as I discussed above, I encourage

---

2   Note that in *Attachment Disability Volume 1,* page 218, I add a third form: persistent self-criticism, a psychological phenomenon, signified by italics: *depression.*

individuals and their loved ones or other supporters to clarify, if possible, their use of the word "depression" in reporting problems. I explain the idea is for them to focus on the underlying reality; that is, the behaviors and feelings they lump into the term.

For example, a not uncommon description of "depression" is "a black cloud coming over me." Typically a careful analysis of the circumstances reveals that the "black cloud" is actually the sudden onset of free-floating anxiety, sometimes described as "a feeling of impending doom." To be sure, clarification of this sort is not accomplished in one or two visits. The idea is to establish this as a goal of management.

Distinguishing Death Preoccupation from Suicidal Intent

Case Study: Lindsey— To Suicide or Not

Lindsey has come to me seriously contemplating Camus' "fundamental question of life"—to suicide or not—and Hamlet's "To be or not to be."

"Yes, I do think about hurting myself, a fair amount—I think especially about cutting. I never do it, though."

I nod and wait for her to fill the silence.

"And yes, I think about suicide sometimes, as I'm sure you read in my therapist's notes. Death by freeway is what I imagine. There's an overpass on my way to school. It looks like the fence would be easy to get over. Speed limit is sixty-five but people do eighty all the time. There wouldn't be time to stop. I think about getting drunk and then climbing up there and jumping off."

"Have you had this thought recently?"

"Yeah …" She reconsiders. "Actually, now that I think about it, not that recently. Maybe a couple weeks? I think I'm better with that prescription they gave me at the crisis center. Those meds seem to work. They calm me down."

Lindsey is a twenty-three-year-old law student who also works part time as a personal care attendant. She has been referred to me by her therapist for follow-up on her medications. She's had eight sessions to date with the therapist, and each has reported to me that they're making progress.

But Lindsey's progress is relative. Her freeway fantasies are less frequent—that's a relief—but she is experiencing a host of other forms of distress. Low energy, difficulty concentrating, reduced appetite. Critical self-talk is a constant, and she expresses hopelessness that this particular problem will ever improve. This pattern of disparaging herself has been with her since the age of sixteen when she discovered a beloved teacher and mentor, a guiding light in her life, was having an affair. Given her age and stage of psycho-sexual development, she was very vulnerable, and her broken trust gave way to anger at herself for ever being a believer—in anything.

The harmful self-talk had become much more intense eight months ago. It was at that point that her recurring thoughts of self-harm escalated to fantasies of suicide.

"What was happening around eight months ago?"

"Oh, I don't know exactly. It's not like there was one certain event. But I know I'd gotten to a point in my relationship with my boyfriend where I realized it was screwed up. I should say *I* was screwed up. I was so clingy. I wanted him around all the time, even though I knew he needed some time to himself. So then he kind of drew back into his shell, and when he wouldn't talk to me, I didn't know how to interpret that. Was he sick or something? Maybe seeing somebody else and scared to tell me?

"It got bad. I remember I texted him one time and he didn't text me back for an hour. I was out of my mind, panicky, thinking maybe something happened to him. Turned out he had just walked to the store and back and forgot to take his phone.

"I hate being like that, so needy. It's disgusting. Finally, I broke up with him."

I nod again and add to my notes: "big boundary issues."

"Back to the sense of hopelessness you mentioned. Do you have any particular spiritual beliefs? Are there certain spiritual practices you engage in?"

"No, my spiritual beliefs are pretty much nonexistent."

"Okay. So the *hopelessness* is a concern to me, because it's one of the four prerequisites to suicide. You're also at risk for another one, opportunity. You tell me you drive past that opportunity every day. The two others, intent and deficient support, are absent for you, fortunately.[3] It's for this reason that I'm not going to recommend you be hospitalized. Hospitals are for emergencies, not 'life issues,' and that's what you're describing.

"However, if you ever start to feel like you're losing control, that's the time to get to a hospital. Don't even wait to talk to me—just go. Tell them to examine you and then call me. You'll probably be feeling better by the time you get there anyhow."

I continue, now less directly and personally, in fact a bit didactically to maintain some distance. I offer the opinion that her "life issue" appears to be a boundary problem, a kind of confusion about whose needs are primary in a relationship. I suggest that now is the time to be patient and sort things out in therapy and continue her medications. I tell her I'd like to see her again in two weeks.

When next we meet, she tells me she has read a book on codependence—a good sign that she's looking at boundary problems. Then, suddenly, she spontaneously confesses that she is a perfectionist.

This gives me an opening for a (again, somewhat arm's length) discussion of the "what if" thoughts that typically drive perfectionism, and I suggest she look into a behavior therapy technique called Exposure/Response Prevention. This will give her some practice in countering her hidden belief that she can control her life, prevent disaster, and banish the pain of life by being "perfect."

---

3   These four prerequisites will help you distinguish death preoccupation from suicidal intent, #2 on the list of the three most important forms of clarification that opened this chapter.

This time I suggest she return in a month, but she's back two weeks later.

"I'm more suicidal than ever. The worst was last Wednesday. But then I stopped taking the Prozac, and things have been fine the past few days."

I note that she had increased her dosage of Prozac, and tell her that could indeed have been a factor in the escalation of suicidal thoughts.

"You know what?" Lindsey offers. "What happened on Wednesday, that was different from how it usually happens. Usually when I think about killing myself I'm alone, late at night. This time it was the middle of the day and I was with people."

I note that this is a very significant observation, a new variable that needs tracking, but I don't want to lose momentum in clarifying issues of perfectionism.

"Interesting," I say before redirecting the conversation. "Since our last session, have you thought at all about the idea I put forth—that perfectionism is a way to deny the suffering that is inherent in living, for which no one is to be blamed?

"But if there's pain, somebody is at fault for that," she disagrees.

"No, not true," I counter. "To be human is to experience pain."

"No, *that's* not true," she insists. "Pain happens in relationships because somebody does something hurtful. If I cause somebody pain, that's my fault, and I should be punished for it. Maybe suicide should be my punishment."

"Look, Lindsey, anyone with half a brain has thought about suicide, and you have more than half a brain. Sooner or later everyone wonders if life is worth living."

Lindsey lowers her eyes and sits in stony silence, giving me and my argument the cold shoulder. The silence continues for an uncomfortably long time.

I finally interject, "My goodness, you are a stubborn one."

After a beat, she bursts into laughter, which breaks the tension. "You've got that right!"

As the session draws to a close, I counsel Lindsey to continue to stay away from the Prozac. I suggest she take the other medication as needed and follow up with her new counselor.

"Come back when you feel like you need to," I conclude.

Two weeks later, she fails to show up for an appointment.

I have had no word from her in the five years since.

Did Lindsey kill herself? If she had, I would have heard about it. Saint Paul is, after all, a largish small town. A death by a fall from an overpass is always reported in the media, and suicide is always considered. The medical examiner routinely asks family, friends, and physicians about signs of suicidal intent. So Lindsey is still out there, dealing with life's pain.

What Can Lindsey Teach Us?

According to Wikipedia, Hamlet's *to be or not to be* musings on the pains of life and the temptation of suicide "is one of the most widely known and quoted lines in modern English, and the soliloquy has been referenced in innumerable works of theatre, literature and music." In other words, Lindsey is not alone in the midst of her suffering. Her preoccupation with tossing herself off a freeway overpass does not mean she is mentally ill. Her misery simply means she is human. And as a human being, she not only is blessed/cursed with awareness, as we all are, but she is also insightful: her experiences tell her she could be hurt again if she reaches out. Escape is imperative. But life's more common escape techniques—marijuana, other drugs, sex, busyness—have not worked for her. Which leaves suicide as the only, ultimate answer.

We usually buttress ourselves against the assaults of life's crises with some combination of social support or spiritual belief. We all face—indeed may have faced—the inevitable anxieties of life's separations and abandonments, as Dr. Kolb once memorably instructed me. We can understand why Lindsey's social support is shaky: her damaged trust. The anxiety-reducing protectiveness of trust is not available to her, nor is, presumably, the solace of belief.

However, we must question her report that her spiritual beliefs are "pretty nonexistent." In fact, she is very spiritual and highly moral. It's just that she believes only in damnation, not salvation or forgiveness or mercy. Only suffering counts, and suffering is her fault because either she causes it or does not rectify it when she encounters it. Her decision to work as a personal care attendant is not a surprise, but it is risky. Anyone in a health care profession knows that when it comes to relief of pain and suffering, demand always exceeds supply.

So, how do we provide protection in a situation such as this? We challenge erroneous beliefs—tactfully of course, but directly. Hence, *Anyone with half a brain thinks about suicide now and then, and you have more than half a brain. Sooner or later everyone wonders if life is worth living.*

In other words, while suicidal thinking may be a sign of mental illness, it may also be a sign of mental awareness; that is certainly true here. Notice that I addressed her unmistakable intelligence, in effect an honest spoonful of sugar to make the bitter medicine go down.

This interpretation served a host of related issues. There was no question that the anxiety associated with her boundary conflicts induced a progressive paralysis; hence treatment with psychotropics was indicated. A much more critical issue, however, was her growing awareness that no relationship is conflict free, that a clash of needs is inevitable even with two loving individuals. This was at odds with her perfectionist belief that she could control suffering if she did things "just right." In other words, to live is to suffer—probably Camus' point—and suffering would always be her "fault"; thus her suicidal ruminations and planning. Indeed, experts comment that psychic pain is a common theme in suicide notes.

You may also wonder, as do I, why my comment about her stubbornness made such a difference. I think

I was responding to her ability to resist, indicating that she was not altogether powerless, that she had strength in the midst of her sense of helplessness, an inner invulnerability and intelligence that she could rely on to guide her through the uncertainties of her life. She felt validated and was able to lower her guard.

In truth, there was really no reason for Lindsey to return to me. She had a therapist lined up, plus a new job to engage her that suited her personality by giving her the opportunity to provide to others the care and comfort that were lacking in her childhood. Hopefully she would experience some healing of her attachment issues without becoming too entangled.

Moreover, I suspect that the sudden collapse of her resistiveness at our third meeting was in retrospect somewhat disturbing, stirring up conflicts of becoming dependent; that was why I left things open-ended at the end of the session. And she has a lot to think about, in fact a lifetime's worth, because the meaning of suffering-midst-existence is never really settled. But she is in a good place to start on that journey.

Identifying the Fears That Lurk Behind Anger

Anger and fear, apparently polar opposites, are actually different manifestations of one underlying dynamic: concerns about separation and loss. Another way to conceptualize this is to think of anger and fear as the energies associated with unmet needs. People suffering from Attachment Disability fear to assert their needs because they anticipate, based on experience, retaliation that could range from cold-shoulder rejection to outright abandonment. So they inhibit their assertiveness and seethe at the injustice of it all.

Thus when a patient's anger is apparent, I have learned to search for their underlying fear. And vice versa: where fearfulness dominates the picture, I think of hidden anger. Come to think of it, this dynamism is an obvious corollary of Dr. Kolb's dictum regarding anxiety: "It's all due to separation."

Recall that Lindsey reports much anxiety but little if any anger. If we are to follow Dr. Kolb's dictum and its corollary, her anxiety is a signal of pressing separation and abandonment concerns resulting from her unmet needs for comfort and protection. She despises these needs because they make her feel weak and vulnerable, and she turns to alcohol and other substances, which only incite more self-loathing. Hence the anger associated with her anxiety is deflected inward, and this elicits the belief that she deserves punishment. Why can't she just be happy and satisfied? But asserting and attending to her unmet needs would surely be too dangerous; such behavior risks the retaliation and punishment that she considers an inevitable part of life. So when the energy associated with her unmet needs begins to worm its way into her consciousness, she panics. Fortunately, her tentative solution—suicide—is so alarming that she risks seeking help.

My insistence that pain not only is part of life but is no one's fault releases some of Lindsey's anger in the form of stubborn denial. When I recognize her stubbornness, which she knows she is feeling, and communicate that I am not offended by her forthright assertiveness, I validate her anger. If pain is part of being human, so is anger—and one of its myriad forms, stubbornness. Hopefully this will set the stage for further exploration of these issues with her therapist.

A similar dynamic is true of Rebecca, fortunately without the suicide scenario. Her anger also boils and seethes, panicking her into a state of paralysis (her "depression") when it threatens to vent, but without evoking a desperate search for relief.

In short, the apparent dichotomy of fear versus anger is a misconception: both are present. I have found that patients more easily accept the notion of this duality when their anger is foremost. Generally their lurking fears of separation and abandonment are not that hidden. But working with fearful and timid souls is a different matter. Their denial is tenacious, yet their anger and its perceived dangerousness must be addressed.

Here is an indirect technique to approach the dynamic:

Dr. C: Having taken a history, pondering it, then says, "You know, I have found that people who are fearful frequently have hidden angers."

Patient: "What do you mean?"

Dr. C: "Well, because of how they have been criticized or punished, they have learned to stuff how they truly feel."

Patient: Silent, obviously considering the idea.

Dr. C. "I'm wondering if that might be the case with you."

Patient: Either affirms or denies, typically the latter.

Dr. C. If the former, "Well, fill me in." If the latter, "Well, it's something to think about, but now let's go on."

A more direct technique is to wonder about the person's life experiences with anger. Was their childhood one of an angry, vengeful parent? Or a household of a terrifying parental cold-shoulder rejection to temper tantrums? In time I lead up to this interpretation: "In other words, in your experience, anger kills ... either you or someone else is destroyed?" Occasionally what then emerges is the memory of a nurturing figure, in response to a display of defiance or stubbornness, clutching her chest while gasping, "Oh, you'll be the death of me!" A few patients, on the other hand, will respond to such probing by dropping out of treatment. Most, however, continue to deny any connection and change the subject, so I postpone further discussion of the issue until later.

Your Takeaways

Healing is like walking up a spiral, building on what you have learned as you climb.

▲

To distinguish "depression" from anxiety, it can be helpful to suggest the individual use the word "worried" instead of "depressed."

▲

Never accept an individual's self-report uncritically.

▲

Clarifying questions can be experienced as intrusive or rejecting; timing is critical.

▲

Search for distortions of your message and be prepared to restate it.

▲

Management of Attachment Disability involves teaching people to learn to *describe* their suffering with less *judging* of it.

▲

Anxiety is an *emotion*; "depression" is *cognitive*, an error in judgment when people blame themselves for the paralysis caused by anxiety.

▲

Suicidal thinking accompanies hopelessness; extreme hopelessness is lethal.

▲

Anger and fear are different manifestations of one underlying dynamic: concerns about separation and loss. Both are energies associated with unmet needs.

▲

Once people understand the grip of their own attachment issues, they will develop their own explanation for why they are gripped.

6

Management Principle #2:

Acceptance

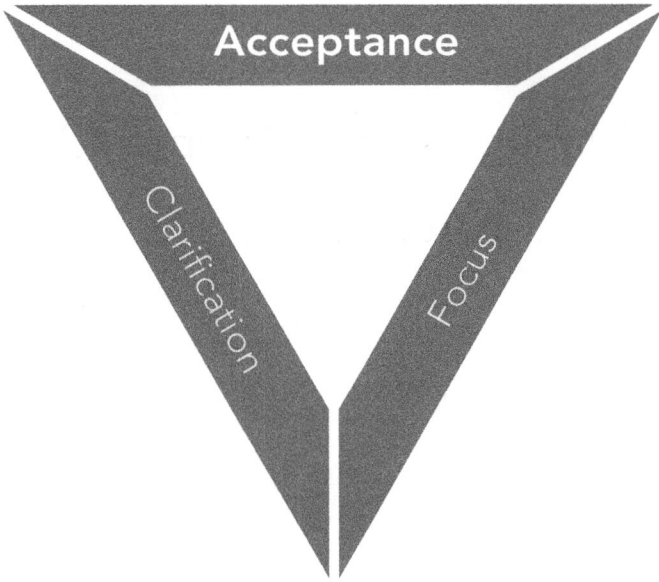

Under any circumstances, experiencing trauma undermines trust. It erodes your confidence in yourself, in others, and in the predictability of life. You search for a cause, and you wonder: *Whose fault is it? Mine? Someone else's? Society's?* You are tempted to blame, which somehow seems "easier" than accepting responsibility, and the adult in you struggles to process the turmoil of blame versus responsibility.

If you are younger or less experienced, your struggles are more intense. The voice of fault seems to echo without end, especially if at the time you were traumatized you were also told it was your fault, that you "deserved" it. So you buy "the blame for the pain."

What you need is a balancing dose of FUBAR.

Life Is FUBAR

It's hard to imagine any kind of trauma that is more intense than combat. Beginning on the first day of boot camp, military training manages the intensity by trust-building. Veterans I know—professionals, patients, friends—tell me you are taught that your buddy "will have your back."

On the other hand, there is what is called the "fog of war"; that is, the uncertainties and contradictions of military leadership. As World War II GIs assessed the fog, they coined the term FUBAR: F***Up Beyond All Recognition. In other words, don't expect logic, or that everything will be under control: just follow orders and commands. In the Navy, say my friends, the acronym for the same wisdom was SNAFU—Situation Normal: All F***UP.

As much as we would like it to be so, life is not predictable. We expect things will change, of course, but our expectations include the notion that a certain amount of what happens in life is foreseeable. Sooner or later, however reluctantly, we come to accept that this will not always be so. But if you are a trauma survivor, acceptance is much more difficult.

Think of Lindsey's iron rule: *if there is pain, someone is guilty.* Her life task is learning to accept that pain is an inevitable part of any relationship. She is certainly responsible for dealing with it because it is *her* suffering; it belongs to her and no one else. But this does not mean she is at fault, that she is worthy of blame. Her feeling of guilt is a false signal, echoes of which will probably always linger. She needs to learn to balance it with another message:

"No blame for the pain."

This is the essence of acceptance. Here is another example: Julie.

Case Study: Julie— The Dangers of Recovery

"Of *course* it's my fault that I'm hurting," Julie says moments into our first session.

"How do you figure that?" I asked.

"I should never have married Glen. I shouldn't have fallen in love with him in the first place. It's because I loved him so much, that's why the hurting never stops."

Julie has been in terrible pain for nearly two years, ever since her young, athletic husband collapsed and died while playing hockey, just eight months into their marriage. The grief that followed was so intense that she lost a dangerous amount of weight and became unable to function. She remained entirely incapacitated for eighteen months, despite continuous and exhaustive psychiatric treatment, including three hospitalizations (one after having been committed following an overdose), a course of electroshock therapy, and trials of six different Antidepressants. Finally, a few months prior to my seeing her, she found a therapist who gained her trust. That therapist had referred her to me with the idea that I could restart her on one of the Antidepressants that had worked in the past.

As I read over Julie's history prior to sitting down with her, a pattern emerged. Over the course of all of those psychiatric interventions, whenever one of them seemed to be making a difference for her, she stopped complying with it. If a drug or a combination of drugs started to help, the pills wound up in the trash.

Her history signaled that she had found a way to blame herself for her anguish, and it was the reason I had opened our conversation by directly asking if her suffering was her "fault." If her history had been less clear yet I suspected self-blame, I might make a "wondering" comment instead, such as "You know, I've been wondering if you might be blaming yourself." Not all expressions of fault are signaled so clearly. Usually self-blame is conveyed indirectly through a slumped posture or an apologetic gesture or tone of voice. A few self-blaming patients, like Maya in the preceding chapter, have even apologized to me when a medication I prescribed for them didn't work, as though a disappointing detour in the search for the most effective drug—which not uncommonly involves some trial and error—could somehow be their fault.

Julie's strategy of rejecting treatment that was working was effective, in that it protected her from the risks of the relationships that health and recovery would inevitably bring into her life. But this "solution" carried a huge cost. She was unable to function because of persistent but unwitting anxiety that the next person she trusted would also drop dead ... and again the loss and grief would be her fault, because once again she had foolishly given her trust to another. In essence, her self-blaming paralyzed her.

Unmanaged Attachment Issues Linger

This vignette, brief as it is, illustrates the role guilt plays in perpetuating attachment issues. While her disability was profound and even life-threatening on occasion, the attachment conflicts driving it were never addressed, and so she remained vulnerable to relapse.

Not all relapse is due to noncompliance, however. Not infrequently it is caused by changing medications. Or it may be precipitated by a new stressful event, welcome or unwelcome: for example, a new romantic interest, or being passed over for a promotion. But Julie's relapse was clearly related to her discontinuing otherwise successful treatment, since "improvement" symbolized once again risking attachment and abandonment. To regain a state of health was *dangerous*; to be disabled was *safe*. Even effective medications could not address her underlying and persisting vulnerability: fears of loss and abandonment. Her guilt lingered.

Adolescents are susceptible to the same dynamic, but it is the rare youngster who can articulate this issue as clearly as Julie did. Ordinarily a pattern of success and relapse like this seems mysterious; "self-defeating" is how we are tempted to label it. But we need to consider the possibility that for some individuals, success signifies danger, danger that will cause pain, and the pain will be their fault. It truly feels safer to fail.

Developing Trust

Such fears of connectedness may be difficult to comprehend if your own ability to attach has not been devastated by trauma and loss of trust. Of course, we have all suffered the stresses of change and have experienced the loss of beloved figures. But in some circumstances perhaps your trust was tested. If you recall how that felt, it takes little imagination to understand the devastation of Julie's loss and her reluctance to move forward, and to appreciate the Catch-22 of her recovery: if she was good at trusting, she probably would not have been sitting in a therapist's office to begin with. She would have learned to accept pain without blame.

Fortunately for Julie, she finally connected with a therapist who, recognizing her fears of recovery, helped her work through them. What was her therapist's magic? This is a vital issue since all trauma victims and their therapists face this dilemma. As a therapist, counselor, or other supportive guide, how do you promote trust?

Let me respond with a story.

Toward the end of my psychiatric training, several of us were wrapping up a psychotherapy seminar with one of our professors, an eminent psychoanalyst. He had struggled for a year to polish our therapy techniques. Once a month we would gather at his mid-Manhattan office and take turns presenting an update on our therapeutic (mis)adventures, offering critiques of our own and the others' performance. When things got murky and one of us would start to flounder, the professor provided clarification and suggestions. By year's end the proceedings were informal and relaxing. We had all bonded and we all knew we were going to graduate; it was, in fact, rather relaxing to pile into a car and go for a ride downtown to his office while taking a break from our official responsibilities as senior residents. Indeed our final meetings were more like a conversation among equals, with him sharing his views on the wider world of psychiatry and psychoanalysis.

During one such audible rumination, he tossed off the comment, "Of course, when it comes to therapy, technique is about twenty percent. The rest is trust, and that is up to you." I remember thinking, *What the #$%&! I wish someone had told me this at the beginning; I would have had a better idea of what I was trying to do!*

Decades later I now realize he was right to a certain extent. For any relationship to flourish, trust is essential, and in most relationship situations—whether personal, parental, or professional—both parties bestow trust to the relationship. Trusting is assumed. But a therapeutic relationship is different. *The disability at the core of Attachment Disability is precisely a wounded ability to trust.* Relationships become dangerous because they create the risk of another abandonment, exploitation, or betrayal, and therapeutic relationships present just this hazard. One of the parties needs to relearn trust, while the other needs to cultivate it. That's what our professor meant: it was our job to promote trusting.

But the ultimate value of his words was lost because he did not cap his months of supervision with a clarifying summary, the gist of which should have been something like "The other eighty percent is knowing when to say something, when to say nothing ... that's how you build trust." That is, as a therapist you can make an incorrect clarification or assessment, but if the timing is right, the person will at least hear it and perhaps, then or later, note anything that doesn't fit. Trust will not be damaged. But if it is mistimed, an otherwise cogent remark will not be accepted. Timing is everything.

Even when our trust has been rebuilt, we can't escape risk, the pain of loss. Acceptance of life's pains requires a touch of FUBAR. To be effective as counselors our task is to gently introduce the notion of FUBAR in a timely fashion.

Recall from chapter 4 that the three principles of management are not sequential. Management is a struggle, a knotted, looping, arduous search of a maze that hopefully will clarify the difference between: 1) the trauma that precipitated the Attachment Disability, and 2) the emotional and cognitive consequences of the disability; that is, the disability about the disability. As denial melts and insight flourishes, it is important to accept the trauma without blame. In other words, as individuals learn to clarify and identify their attachment problems—"owning the pain" in therapist-speak—it is critical they also learn "no blame for the pain." That is, they need support and encouragement to accept the lost trust without searching for an agent to blame for the loss. The "what" of the loss is important, not the "why."

Forgive and Forget?

In a sense *acceptance* addresses the venerable but dubious saying "Forgive and forget." In my view, however, it involves something entirely different: it's "Forgive and *never* forget." Here's why.

Even if we succeed in both forgiving and "forgetting" the trauma—even if we are somehow able to massage our consciousness into a state of amnesia—the potential for disability remains embedded in our neurons. This means that when circumstances later warn of impending trauma, either in fact or imagination, we cannot resort to previously learned adaptive strategies for protection *because we haven't learned any.* Forgetting short-circuits learning, leaving us with no alternative "bag of tricks" to fall back on. Once again we find ourselves more or less helpless, and that is when the temptation to assess blame emerges.

On Blaming

To be sure, blaming has a certain survival function: if projected outward, it creates meaning in a world that otherwise would appear meaningless. Blame permeates our society. Look again at this morning's headlines if you doubt it; you will rarely find a problem without a search for a villain to blame. This is what makes blaming so seductive. It allows society to shift and evade responsibility, to project it onto an external agent. It promotes inertia, which is why it takes a crisis to alter society's trajectory, and it doesn't always happen even then. Or it allows us to justify retaliation and risk overreacting.

Blame can let us shift responsibility for the consequences of our own behavior to someone or something else. Or we look inward. In my years as a psychiatrist I have seen the concept of free-floating anxiety disappear from popular culture, to be replaced by "depression" as the "explanation" of personal problems, as we have discussed. Depression, no matter how painful, is easier to "own" than anxiety because we are told that "depression" is a *disease* and therefore not under our control. But anxiety? That's a different story. Who do we blame but ourselves for what appears to be a moral defect, a lack of willpower?

Two groups of people are especially burdened by blaming: addicts in recovery and individuals with Attachment Disability. In fact, as addicts progress through recovery, it is not uncommon for them to discover that the turmoil of damaged trust, previously "solved" by the use of substances, has not only returned but also threatens to undermine sobriety by promoting craving. Let's examine this commonality.

Blaming Can Undermine Addicts Struggling to Maintain Recovery

One of the functions of the Twelve Steps is to teach addicts to live without blame. Because of two complications, *relapse* and *unhappiness*, this ideal is frequently tested as recovering addicts struggle to maintain their sobriety. It is worth exploring how this works with addiction because the same forces are operating in attachment-disabled people who are struggling with their own version of "recovery"; that is, who are learning, over time, to manage their condition.

Relapse

If addicts in recovery are unable to resist resuming substance use, they undergo "relapse," to use AA lingo. Thereafter, if they are referred to me for consultation, part of my evaluation is to inquire about how the relapse happened. Typically such relapsers rationalize their behavior with a statement something like "Well, since I did it, I must have chosen to do it." They see themselves as having deliberately "chosen" to return to their addiction. In other words, they do not understand the return to using represents a return of out-of-control behavior. To them it feels as if they must have "decided" to use. *It is my fault* is how they typically evaluate their fall from the grace of sobriety. They still do not understand the First Step; that is, that they are out of control and must turn to a higher power.

In fact, a relapse is not a "choice" but a reflection of an inability to exercise an alternative, to find a different way of dealing with the trauma-induced turmoil of damaged trust. There is nothing else to fall back on. True, the relapser's choices are "voluntary" in the sense that their behavior originated in and proceeded from themselves and no one other than themselves. But this does not mean they were capable of exercising "will power" to perform an alternate behavior that would defuse the impulse to return to their addiction. Their behavior was voluntary—it was their "choice" in the sense that they were the agents of their behavior—but not their "choice" in the sense that they had more options among which to choose. Their "choice," in short, was *voluntary but not free.*

This is why the first of the Twelve Steps refers to powerlessness and calls for turning to a higher power. And this is why Alcoholics Anonymous and other recovery organizations urge addicts to attend groups and find a sponsor; that is, to learn the behavior of asking for help when in need. If addicts learn this one new trick, this one new solution, namely surrounding themselves with a network of sober—and (hopefully) non-blaming—peers to turn to when craving flares up, the odds of maintaining sobriety are significantly improved.

The Addiction–Attachment Disability Parallel

It is important to understand addiction because the repetitive, self-destructive behavior that is the dominant and perplexing characteristic of addicted individuals is very similar to the behavior of attachment-disabled individuals. Both seem unable to extract themselves from its power even with help. The patterns of behavior, in my experience, are highly correlated because as addicts recover, they not infrequently report trauma, from which substances provide relief.

Addiction is the result of at least three processes.

First of all, it involves a form of learning called "*con-

ditioning"—both classical (Pavlovian) and operant (Skinnerian)—that all of us experience as we act on and react to our environment, especially our social environment, and most especially those figures in our social environment who are poised to recognize, reward, frustrate, or punish our behavior: parents, sponsors, friends, teachers, and so on. We thus undergo reinforcement as certain behaviors and associated needs are recognized (positive reinforcement) while other behaviors and associated needs are ignored (negative reinforcement). Both processes involve multiple complex feedback loops.

Second, both repetitive (training and coaching) and solo (so-called "one-shot learning") conditioning can produce *physical changes in our neuron connections*, which can favor certain responses becoming more likely than others. This is how we learn to drive, play a sport, fit in, and respond to social and environmental cues, among many other things. Our nervous and muscular systems become "grooved" and strengthened, creating a probability that subsequent similar cues will elicit similar, even automatic responses; in other words, what we call "habits." Once so deeply engrained, habits are difficult to resist. In short, as we learn, our tissues and cells change physically.

But addictive behavior rests on a third factor: blunting of the hypothalamic-pituitary-adrenal axis response to stress and anxiety. It is thought that this provokes craving and predisposes one to relapse. In fact studies of early life stress tend to predict later alcohol and drug dependence. In consequence, the addicted and/or attachment-disabled individual's ability to choose is restricted when confronted with stress-induced cues. This illustrates how complex the notion of choice is.

It is this very conditioned neuron "grooving" that makes overcoming both addiction and Attachment Disability so difficult. To be sure, such individuals do retain a limited capacity to exercise choice. For example, they can elect to participate in a supportive environment such as a treatment center or a sober house or a group home, in the hope that they will undergo "counter-conditioning" to refurbish their ability to choose. But the traumatized brain without retraining is a brain with an impoverished capacity to exercise choice when it comes to a confrontation, either direct or symbolic, with trauma residuals.

There is a mystery here. We know that some trauma victims do recover, somehow escape their paralysis. They do regain the ability to be decisive and "choiceful"; for example, to choose not to drop out of treatment or counseling when they experience a setback. In such cases, even if I have the opportunity to develop more detail, I find I never fully understand why things began to take a turn for the better. It always seems easier to reconstruct why things fall apart versus why they improve. Let's just chalk this up as a more specific example of the mystery of learning. That is, to paraphrase the old saying, non-learning has many parents; learning is an orphan. Here is where the alert counselor, recognizing a shift in attitude and motivation, steps up with counter-conditioning. You stay silent in the face of maladaptive behaviors and comments, hoping they will extinguish, instead gently and tactfully recognizing adaptive maneuvers. Such a modification of an individual's stimulus configuration rearranges their synaptic junctions within the central nervous system. Those that facilitate maladaptive behavioral and cognitive habits begin to wither while neuronal connections serving the more adaptive habits are strengthened. We will address this at greater length in the next chapter on focus.

For example, I have found that many addicts who are apparent nonresponders to treatment actually have never gone beyond the First Step due to a maladaptive habit of introjecting blame. Not truly understanding their out-of-control state, they ascribe their out-of-controlness to "*my fault*" rather than "*my powerlessness.*" Seemingly accepting the "blame" for their relapse, they actually are avoiding responsibility for it. To fully acknowledge they have no power over their behavior involves a loss of self-esteem that is too threatening to face.

There is a lesson here for all of us. As parents and teachers and therapists and physicians, we must resist the impulse to blame when our children and students and patients fail to learn or get well. And it is a certainty that we in the helping and teaching professions, and we parents as well, will face this crisis of powerlessness. For there will always be the student who will not learn, the patient who will not heal, the inebriate who will relapse, the child who will not conform. But this is not forever, just for today. So it is important for us to recognize that all power is limited, and learn to accept without panicking or blaming that we are powerless … for now.

Unhappiness

Apart from blaming themselves for relapses, addicts in recovery can also be tripped up by blaming themselves for not feeling happy despite achieving sobriety. The same is true for attachment-disabled people who have made some progress in therapy or counseling, who have achieved clarity about their condition and have begun to accept it

In fact, we are not to be blamed for being unhappy: after all, life is FUBAR. But it is one thing to be unhappy and quite another to feel it is our own "fault." Much of therapy consists of employing strategies such as reframing and redirection (see the next chapter) to teach individuals to "own" their problems without blaming themselves or others for those problems. It is not the pain of life that crushes people; it is the blame for the pain. True, we have to accept responsibility for the pain we experience because it is our pain; we are the suffering ones, not someone else. But accepting responsibility is not the same as buying into blame. A critical difference, this, and not infrequently a life preserving one.

Blaming Drives Cutting and Self-Mutilation

Traumatized youngsters and adults are particularly burdened by blaming. Their lives have been scarred by lost or abusive relationships, frequently both. Children are especially vulnerable to interjecting blame when it comes to dealing with the loss of a loving figure. The only way they can comprehend a world in which such a meaningful and powerful entity can completely vanish is to conclude it must have been their fault. So they cling tenaciously to their blame; it provides meaning in a FUBAR world.

Even in the absence of a lost relationship, individuals who have been abused or exploited are especially vulnerable to self-blame because, inevitably, the perpetrator blamed them at the time of the injury. Thus they are double victimized both by the trauma and, what is arguably worse, the responsibility for it. But regardless of age and the type of trauma, the attachment-disabled person's blaming, whether of self or others, is apparent from the get-go in most cases, the exception being an attachment issue of the entangled type. In that case, the blaming is disguised, manifested by cutting and self-mutilation.

Such behaviors, in my experience, are always—always!—a signal of a harsh and vindictive self-critical inner voice that the mutilation is designed to relieve. These suffering adolescents (generally adolescents, with occasional adult exceptions—as people grow to adulthood they usually develop more self-awareness and are less in denial), if they should come to your attention, are deceptive because of their blandness. While the mutilation may seem—and may very well be—a cry for attention, its greater significance is the extremely entangled personality structure beneath the placid, benevolent smile.

These individuals are especially challenged by their sensitivity to others' unhappiness. They come to perceive life as an endless procession of suffering souls needing rescue. They are the "catchers in the rye" out to protect a world of unhappy or demanding parents, relatives, and, particularly, peers.

The sight or even the prospect of a sad or lonely or disappointed expression on a parent's or chum's face is unbearable pain to these sufferers. They are highly motivated to assume the problem-solver/peacemaker role within the family and between peers. They are the "good" student, the "good" child. Not infrequently they become quite adept in this role, which brings satisfaction and smiles to their parents and teachers. This is highly reinforcing for the youngster because it meets their need to please and satisfy others. So the next unhappy face is even more likely to elicit enabling behavior.

But there is always more suffering than they can manage. Slowly but inevitably life appears to verify the cynical statement *Life is hard and then you die*. Life becomes an endless chore of figuring how to make happy a constant parade of unhappy faces. We know, for example, it is precisely from such concerns that so many youngsters with sexual identity and gender issues deal with their problems by concealing them. These children correctly assess the unhappy responses a frank revelation of their doubts and feelings would be likely to provoke, unhappiness that could only be relieved by them promising not to have such doubts and feelings.

Eventually life comes to mean being alone—you can't confide because it will make someone unhappy if you start to complain—or being a slave to the happiness of another.

As these children battle their isolation or servitude, they reveal their suffering in anonymous notes left in public places, or sometimes in quite unambiguous essays in response to school assignments, or sometimes via the more ambiguous signal of self-mutilation.

Such youngsters are uniquely susceptible to the drama of high school life and are at risk of becoming deeply responsible for the miseries of their peers, especially if they cannot rescue them. Peer deaths by suicide or misadventure can elicit echoing self-destructive behaviors. Such extreme sensitivity to the concerns of others complicates their management for it contaminates connections with their teachers, counselors, and therapists. Healthy and secure therapeutic boundaries are a must when you engage such adolescents. Their blank façade is, after all, a defense against allowing you, a stranger, a peek at their unhappiness. You might become concerned, and they don't need another soul worrying about them. So you get stiffed, pleasantly and discreetly to be sure, but stiffed nonetheless.

Hence, when I am referred a youngster for a medication evaluation, I always inquire whether there is a therapist and, if there is, how things are going. *"How is the chemistry between you?"* I ask. If it seems to be okay, I might just nod or, perhaps, make a vague recommendation that they consider working on what strikes me as an unexplored but relevant issue, entanglement or abandonment, for example. But sometimes I find things are not okay. *"He asks too many questions"* or *"She gets too upset when I tell her how I feel, so I just keep quiet."* When I hear this I always take pains to validate the report. I note that the discomforts accompanying any treatment process, whether the problem is physical or mental, are part of owning the problem. Then I clarify that trust is the solvent of effective therapy, and if the youngster and sponsors determine that trust is lacking, they need to consider obtaining a second opinion.

Occasionally the self-mutilation becomes concealed by a façade of acting-out. But such self-injurious behavior is always a tip-off: behind the furor lurks an entangled soul. Recall the situation with Lara (chapter 3), whose cutting was the first sign of her worries about her father's behavior. Would he survive his mania for extreme sport?

Acceptance

Opposed to blaming is the notion of *acceptance*. A stance of acceptance focuses on *what is*, not *why* it is, not what it *should be*. A stance of acceptance seeks facts, not explanations or solutions. Not that the latter are inappropriate inquiries, but inquiry without a solid grip on *what is* slithers into speculation or fantasy. The scholastic philosophers defined truth as *the mind conformed to reality*; they distinguished between the facts and what you make of the facts. To the extent that your thinking conforms to the facts, and only to the facts, to that extent you possess the truth. Facts are "out there"; truth is in your head—which makes fact prior to truth. And one of the most important of all facts is the fact of FUBAR.

We must not conclude, however, that we are somehow diminished or enfeebled by grabbing life's unpredictability by its throat and holding on. To the contrary, a realistic awareness of loss, real or symbolic, impending or distant, unlocks our creative potential because *to accept what can't be replaced means to recognize what can be*. This is what is meant by the old saying "The truth shall set you free."

We recognize what can be changed, and that is where we concentrate our efforts. The truthful mind is a focused mind is an effective mind. So the mantra for us and our patients is this: *accept the problem*. Again, it is not the pain of life that crushes; it is the blame for the pain.

Acceptance Promotes Responsibility

People engaged in learning to manage Attachment Disability must learn to take personal responsibility for their life problems. This does not mean the problems are their "fault"—again, there is no blame—but it does mean they, and only they, will have to live with their issues. Their tasks are both to accept help and to search for something to replace or repair, if possible, their Attachment Disability.

Responsibility Leads to Describing, Not Judging

This, too, is not a self-evident concept. We are moral creatures in the sense that from birth we register both our experience and its significance to our well-being. No experience is processed free of its significance to survival. Human morality begins as the infant's nervous system assigns survival value to the stimulus situations it encounters. By the second year of life, toddlers display a powerful capacity for a primitive but urgent labeling of life's options; that is, what is "good" or "bad" for them. If something is the latter, parents will surely encounter the nightmare that haunts the early years of child care—a red-faced eighteen-month-old screaming, *"Nooooo!"* The task of teaching and parenting is to transmute this energy into an adaptive, resourceful, motivated, considerate, productive human being who takes into account the rights and needs of others when evaluating the goodness and badness—that is, the moral dimensions—of its actions.

Of course, we all know this is not always how things work out, as the need for this handbook demonstrates.

Thus the commonplace observation that adolescents have a keen sense of the rightness and wrongness of things. Attachment-disabled adolescents bring to school the same moral keenness. Unfortunately they do not bring with them a modulated, balanced moral sense. It tends to be harsh and punitive and judgmental, no doubt a reflection of their nurturing or lack of thereof. Their moral filter is crude and extreme, especially when it comes to how they feel and think. Thoughts, feelings, and emotions are never experienced as such: in isolation. Instead they are experienced with a moral valence, an overpowering sense of goodness or badness.

Our task is to rebalance the inner life of youngsters and adults alike by teaching them how to describe their world without judging the experience. As I tell them, *"You already are pretty good when it comes to opinions about the stuff of your life; let's see now if you can learn to experience the 'stuff' without deciding whether it is good or bad."* Not unexpectedly, since we are dealing here with an engrained life attitude of thought and speech, this is not immediately accomplished. I might first model and reframe for them an example of descriptive language, then use a behavior therapy technique of repetitive prompts and redirection to promote its adoption. I will discuss reframing and redirection in the next chapter.

Your Takeaways

Life is uncertain—but we didn't make life that way.

▲

Own the pain, not the blame. It is not the pain of life that crushes people; it is the blame for the pain.

▲

Forgive but *never* forget.

▲

Choice is always voluntary but not always free.

▲

To accept what can't be replaced means to recognize what can be replaced.

▲

Knowing when to say something and when to say nothing ... that's how therapy builds trust.

▲

A therapist's task is to allow individuals to "own" their suffering while resisting the temptation to "fix" it.

7

Management Principle #3: Focus on What Can Be Changed

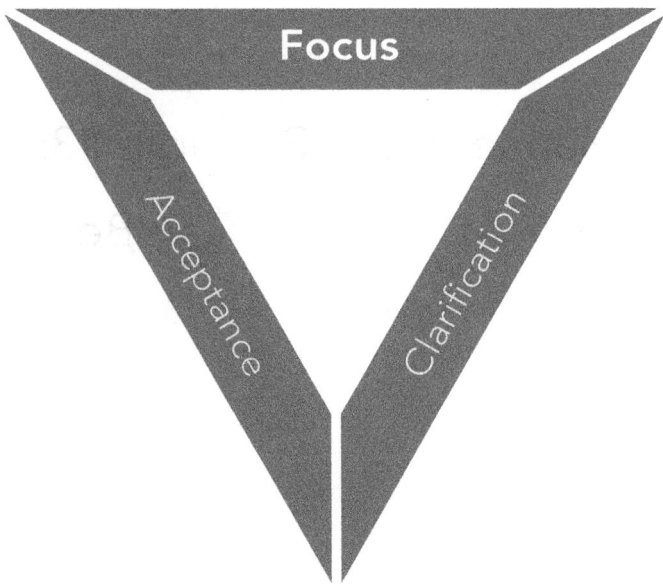

Focus

Acceptance

Clarification

We all know from personal experience that any illness that is acute or chronic is associated with some form of disability; disease and disability go together. As the song goes, "You can't have one without the other." If we are fortunate, we learn to tolerate our dependency on others during the period of disability while we wait for treatment, rehabilitation, and Mother Nature to heal our disease and its residuals. In other words, we focus on what we can change—right now, today—while tolerating what we can't change.

Things become murky, though, if the disability occurs as a result of trauma and there is no notable disease process. Commonly in these cases you will encounter attachment issues in disguise; that is, Attachment Disability *consequences*: constant worries, unhappy relationships, "depression" or pain that does not respond to medications, unsatisfying work, inexplicable irritability, repetitive failures, clawing guilt, and more, alone or in combination.

In working with someone whose disability stems from trauma, you start with clarification, as we saw in the first chapter on managing Attachment Disability. And if things go well, previously disguised or unacknowledged attachment issues may emerge. Assuming that the individual is also learning how to accept the pain of trauma with less blame, the next step is to identify what the person can change in his or her life and establish this as the focus of a treatment plan.

*Learning a new bag of tricks is
the ultimate goal*

(Let me remind you these steps are sequential only in handbooks like this, not in "real life." In a counseling or therapy setting, they are fluctuating shapes in the fog of counseling that will, if all goes well, take on substance and clarity.)

Two Techniques to Change Attachment Disability: Reframing and Redirection

Attachment-disabled people will come to you because they are having personal, school, or work challenges. Helping them remedy this involves two (again, not necessarily sequential) techniques: *reframing* and *redirection*. The idea of reframing is to *identify* a target disability that is susceptible to change. Redirection involves maintaining *focus* on the targeted disability and not becoming distracted by subordinate issues that can't be changed … right now, today.

I have encountered formal treatment plans that cite and attempt to address multiple problems simultaneously; on one occasion I counted as many as thirteen.

But rather than adopting such a scattershot approach, I find the odds of success are much improved if you address the one issue that seems most susceptible to change and maintain a steady aim on that. I have discovered that if I am fortunate and that problem starts to crumble, other problems have a way of dissolving as well.

Identifying susceptibility to change includes its inverse: identifying *in*susceptibility to change. Some life issues are not immediately responsive to the tools you can offer. A wider support system may be required; for example, housing or legal or child-care assistance. Here the goal would be to identify the need and arrange a referral and then suggest a follow-up to see how things are working out. If there is some resistance to seeking help, or a failure to follow through, this would suggest an underlying issue with shame about, guilt about, or fear of seeking help. And that might well be the basic disability.

Reframing

Again it is important to recognize that the three management techniques of *clarification*, *acceptance*, and *focus* are not consecutive. Rather, they are intertwined, which means that inevitably your therapeutic work will be a mixture of all three, hoping to identify and target a disabling issue susceptible to modification without the distractions of blaming. Now and then you will need to remind your clients that the world is FUBAR. And you will also want to emphasize that in a FUBAR world *it is a serious error to wait for other parties or events to change.* Change will inevitably occur, but the idea is not for the individual to passively wait to see how things turn out, but to focus on how they themselves might do things differently.

We can use as an example of reframing a scenario we visited in the last chapter: those struggling to maintain sobriety.

Usually there is a history of relapse and multiple unsuccessful treatment experiences. With such individuals I avoid what might be a more conventional approach, such as trying to identify relapse triggers or encouraging a return to AA participation. Instead I ask, *What's in it for you to stay sober? Why be sober?*

The question flips the script, shifting the focus from doing what might keep others happy—people like probation officers, family, or friends—to doing what might make the disabled individual happy. Will staying clean be good for them? Is this trip necessary? I might point out that if there is little in it for them, even should they achieve sobriety they won't be happy. They will feel trapped by someone else's wishes, which is bound to create resentment: what AA refers to as a "dry drunk." Of course, we live in a society, and to get by we must on occasion please others. But we must also pay attention to our own needs and satisfactions. Sometimes I paraphrase the Second Greatest Commandment: other-love doesn't work without self-love.

On occasion I will even pop the *What's in it for you?* question—that is, I will reframe—with patients who are currently successful at sobriety to help their focus remain aligned with their needs.

In short, the idea is to identify and frame a target

behavior that is susceptible to modification. For example, I suggested that Helen think of herself as "fearful" rather than "depressed," also that she learn to be her "own doctor" when it came to figuring out which of her medications were needed. With Georgina the target was helping her mother deal with her impending graduation by reassuring her she was a "good enough" mother. The focus with Rebecca was similar to Helen's: think of herself as "worried" rather than "depressed," and to focus on what she "needed" to do rather that what she "should" do.

Redirection

Simply identifying a behavior to be modified will not, of course, modify the behavior. Neither Helen nor Georgina nor Rebecca did this simply because I said so. They needed coaching and training to acquire and develop the more adaptive habit. Which is what counseling, reduced to its essentials, is all about: learning. Helen and Georgina and Rebecca all needed *redirection*.

Here are some other common Attachment Disability behaviors, along with examples of how you might redirect these behaviors—adding a new trick to the individual's bag.

Habitual Apologizing

Many attachment-disabled people go through life continually apologizing and self-blaming whenever things don't work out as expected. This is extremely disabling because to blame is to *surrender power*. Then, having rendered themselves helpless, they end up waiting for some external force to either forgive or punish them, typically a mixture of both. If forgiven, they will feel rescued. If punished, that will feel familiar, and thus paradoxically safe. But safety comes at a price: reinforcement of their belief that their problems are their own fault.

Even worse is their not learning from experience that the next time they might want to try a different way of dealing with the issue; they have lost the opportunity to discover a new trick for their bag of resources with which to manage their disability. The hidden cost of unrealistic apologizing is dooming yourself to a life that offers little satisfaction and happiness.

Recall Maya from chapter 5, whose mantra was "Everything is my fault." In our previous meetings I had noticed and remarked on this very habitual but unrealistic world view that she was to blame for everything, commenting that, in fact, life truly is FUBAR. *Look at the morning headlines*, I told her, *watch the evening newscast. Some things in life are just awful and have nothing to do with you.*

Although one trial of rather rudimentary behavior modification—modeling assertive language—seemed ineffective then, if used consistently I have seen powerful effects with "depressed" patients; for example, individuals who have tried meditation, self-hypnosis, or progressive relaxation without benefit. Sufferers need to be reminded that no therapeutic technique is a hundred percent effective. So it will be necessary to repeat this redirective prompting if the habit of self-blaming is particularly entrenched, as it often is when the disability is related to attachment issues.

Here is another related technique I find useful. After a patient makes a statement with an implied—typically through a change in posture or tone of voice—or an actual self-critical assessment, you can encourage them to say the same thing but without an apology. *"Let's see if you can say that without apologizing for what you feel or think or did. Be descriptive, less judgmental."*

Some catch on quickly while others may be puzzled, confused, even irritated, unaware of the guilt beneath the message. On such occasions you can call attention to their body language, encourage them to be more forthright, perhaps even model their words back to them more assertively. It is important to match your use of the technique to their ability to tolerate and learn from it, but this is true of all coaching.

Another method is to designate a gesture—perhaps raising my hand in a "hold it" motion or cupping my hand to my ear: "What?"—that I will use to prompt them to reframe an apologetic behavior or statement. And sometimes I supplement this by giving them a prescription to post on their bathroom mirror, such as: *"Describe your life, don't judge it,"* for a daily reminder of the mental state they need to develop. I explain, "You are pretty good at judging the 'goodness' or 'badness' of your thoughts and feelings. Now let's see if you can develop another habit: simply describing them to yourself, 'owning' them in your own mind without labeling them."

The idea is to encourage patients to look at *what* they feel and think with less preoccupation about *how* they feel and think. In order to manage their Attachment Disability, they need to figure out the survival content of their mental activities—to what extent they are concerned with the tasks they must carry out to sustain life, such as securing food and shelter—while avoiding contamination by moral concerns; that is, notions of goodness or badness. They need to distinguish the actual moral world (the world of behavior and its consequences) from the inner moral world, the world of threat and retaliation and separation. The goal is not to erode the capability to make moral assessments—most patients are pretty good at this, perhaps even too good—but to create a cognitive balance by enhancing their capability to make survival assessments as well.

This approach has its limitations. More timid or reserved patients might find both my behavior and the assertiveness I advocate too threatening if they are not prepared for it. Timing is critical. And a few are simply afraid of raising their voice; they fear they might lose control or that others will go out of control. They understand the rationale of the tactic, but to emit assertive vocalizations is threatening. Any hint of energy in their own voice recreates past abuse experiences, so they freeze up.

And with some people their blaming may be so deeply wired in that they may not be conscious of it. Addressing the blaming directly not only sails right over their heads but risks aggravating the problem. Here is yet another situation that, as they appraise it, is their fault. They are so bogged down by anxiety they will simply find this technique incomprehensible. In fact, it will feel like more punishment because their world is always one of fault and retaliation. Such individuals require different management techniques, perhaps play therapy or role playing.

Paralyzing Expectations

People with attachment issues can develop paralyzing anxiety as they encounter the expectations—real or imagined—of support system figures, whether family, friends, or coworkers. Should they comply with their wishes or resist? It seems neither answer is a good one. The former stirs up anger, the latter guilt and fears of abandonment. If there is a notable trauma background, frequently this anxiety-induced paralysis is misinterpreted as "depression" and is accompanied by self-blaming.

Conflicts of this sort are caused by not understanding that dealing with them is a survival issue, not a moral one, and that all "solutions" are a mixture of the acceptable and unacceptable, the foreseen and the unforeseen. In other words, it is important to redirect such clients by reminding them (1) we live in a FUBAR world, (2) conflict-free options are unlikely, and (3) therefore any decision will incorporate a mixture of both guilt and anger. So the issue becomes this: What would be the more tolerable: guilt or anger? I also suggest to them that either emotion will be easier to bear if they view it as something they choose to endure rather than considering it as something imposed on them by an external agent. Also, to redirect the decision making, I recommend replacing the word "should" with the word "need" as they consider their options, as I did with Rebecca. That is, not *What should I do?* but rather *What do I need to do?*

Distrust

Distrust may be quite apparent or it may be buried. Signs of hidden distrust among attachment-disabled individuals include 1) discursive and rambling statements, 2) not listening to the feedback they ask for, and 3) minimizing positive feedback.

Crippling distrust is the primary effect of trauma. Its consequence is a conditioned anticipation of rejection and rebuff. Neutralizing distrust and restoring the ability to trust must be the fundamental focus of counseling.

Distrust is rarely liquidated by the direct approach of earnestly soliciting trust; only the gullible would respond. And I can assure you that by the time a traumatized person walks into your office, all gullibility has been leached away.

Conceivably an effective gambit is to meet distrust head-on. That is, if your client greets you with the challenge, "Why should I trust you?" you might respond with something forthright, for example, "Well, why should you? You hardly know me." Interviews that start like this often turn out to be very interesting and entertaining, because you are actually, as my professors used to say, *talking to the unconscious.* People like this wish to have a relationship but are afraid of one, so this introductory exchange helps establish a comfortable boundary.

Sometimes the distrust is cloaked with anger. The

thing to remember with anger is that it is fear with a different face. Anger and fear are twins; they always go together—where there is one, the other is also present. But they differ in this respect: Generally it is easier to help people tap into the fear behind anger, while doing the reverse is much more difficult. It is easy for the fearful to recognize how they are intimidated by the prospect of others' scorn or anger, much more difficult for them to accept that their fears serve to keep their own furies in check. An angry person is a person who expects to be rejected, discounted, rebuffed, ignored, perhaps even abused. In their experience "help" is a noise that other people make when they are about to exploit or betray them.

Occasionally you might deal with this directly by saying, "Okay, I know you are angry about _____. Now tell me what you are afraid of." Or, "I get the impression you figure I'll be like the other helpers and give you the brush." Sometimes this pays off by going directly to their distrust and abandonment concerns. More often, however, after allowing the personpatients to ventilate emphatically for a while, perhaps an interview or two, you could redirect them as follows: "Let's see if you can repeat what you have just said but in a more conversational, quieter tone." Then you might model the same words or phrases for them.

The idea is that you never, as my professors advised us residents, serve as a punching bag. Playing rope-a-dope may have helped Ali win fights, but therapy is not a contest with a winner and a loser. Rather, it is a learning situation for both, where there is every reason to believe that both parties can "win" as the therapist learns from the patient, and the patient from the therapist.

Rambling

Verbosity you could characterize as rambling has many causes: mania, psychosis, manipulation, dementia, attentional deficiencies, or some combination thereof. But the most common is an underlying Attachment Disability with marked abandonment concerns. These unhappy people are driven by a need to get everything in before the meeting ends because, in their experience, there is no guarantee of another. They have learned relationships with support professionals are fragile; they can disappear overnight without warning, especially in our modern era of group rather than solo practice and annual changes in insurance coverage. They have developed what we therapists call "rejection sensitivity."

But it does not serve their interests to allow them to endlessly ramble and digress. If the so-called "talking therapy" is to be beneficial, learning must take place. Otherwise it is a waste of time and resources for both parties. Both are frustrated. Patients feel ignored, therapists burned-out. So I cannot overemphasize the importance of what might seem a rather minor behavioral tactic.

For their sake and mine, I manage ramblers with a redirection tactic. After listening for a while, I might make the request, "Let's see if you can boil down what you just said into six words or less." Some are able to do so. In fact a few, after a moment or so of silent concentration, can not only deliver the requested summary but triumphantly tick off each word finger by finger as they do so. Others are perplexed and need help. To them I might say, "Well, in six words is this what you were trying to say?" then make a stab at boiling it down for them.

Of course, I have to manage my own verbosity as well. The idea is to tailor my statement to fit the patient's attention span. Not that I am always successful. To guard against running off at the mouth myself—driven by my own need for attention—from time to time I will ask patients to repeat what I have just said. This focuses the two of us. I clarify that the important thing is for them to hear my feedback, and correct it if it is misinterpreted. Whether it fits or not is another matter; that is up for them to decide. But without listening—and it is my job to promote their ability to listen—they are deprived of the opportunity to learn.

One of the more startling instances of lurking rejection sensitivity is when the feedback is exactly the opposite of what I propose. For example, when I treat chronic pain patients, I include a detailed review of their (often extensive) medical records, which typically reveal no indication that they have a life-threatening condition. After reporting such a conclusion, I've learned to carefully double-check what they heard because often they hear me saying "You mean it's all in my mind!" This is understandable since they've been told before, erroneously, that their problem is "psychological" or "somatoform" when, in fact, the more accurate statement is that the cause of their disabling pain is unknown.

Not Listening

Here people are dominated by a mental cycle of painful worries and concerns related to prior rejections and abandonments. They may seem attentive to inquiries or feedback, but frequently these do not seem to register. Sometimes they are rather unaware of their preoccupation, apologize when it's pointed out to them, and promise to try harder. Others may have more insight, reporting, "My mind doesn't shut down" or "I get distracted." A few may have little to say, clearly distrustful of engagement.

Regardless of the cause, and even when you're dealing with alert and attentive individuals, it is important to be concise and focused when making inquiries and providing feedback. I try to limit my responses to a few sentences at a time—I'm not always successful, I must admit—then pause to see whether and how my words are assimilated. Things do get lost in translation, as they say. This is less likely to occur if you deliver your message in bits and pieces.

Experts in interview technique advise us doctors never to conclude a consult with "Do you have any questions?" This is considered bad form; they maintain it may actually come across as a brusque dismissal. They seem to think that a well performed interview will leave no questions. Of course, only an "expert" could reach such a conclusion. There are always questions: that is our nature for we are, to paraphrase the classical definition of mankind, the questioning animal.

So instead, with a mental genuflection in the direction of correctness, I often manage the ending like this: "I'm going to do something the experts say I should never do. They say I never should ask if there are any questions, so instead I'm going to say 'I'm wondering if you have any questions.'" This usually elicits a laugh and prepares for a smooth closing transition. Or I may say something like, "Well, I'm the one who up to now has been asking questions; now it is your turn."

Minimizing Positive Feedback

People whose rebuffs and rejections have conditioned them to expect more of the same are likely to experience positive feedback as a sugar-coated preliminary to abandonment. They do not seem to "hear" what you say and brush off your feedback as if it never happened.

The critical piece here is to recognize achievement without any subtext implying continuing performance. To do otherwise risks triggering success fears. The message must be "You did well" without the implication "I expect the same from now on." At the same time it is very important now that things have improved for you to resist the impulse to change the treatment protocol; for example, the length or frequency of subsequent visits. Any change would be experienced as a punishment.

If this tactic is properly executed, individuals will experience the recognition they need but feared would not be theirs because of past brush-offs by professionals. On occasion it is possible to directly access such fears with a direct inquiry, such as "Do you ever worry this might be the last time you will have a chance to talk about what is on your mind?"

Habitual Pleasing

Many people with attachment issues have become so adept at detecting and complying with social expectations that they lose sight of their own needs and feelings. A certain amount of social awareness is necessary to get by in life, but when carried to extremes this becomes a profound impairment. Habitual pleasing is a significant cause of the excess disability that will bring many a person to your door. And it can undermine your counseling.

Therefore it is vital that you from time to time unstructure the dialogue by ceding the agenda to the one seeking treatment. To do this, following the opening, housekeeping stage of a session, I might make a statement something like "Well, that brings me up to date ... it looks like we have [X] minutes remaining, so over to you, whatever you would like to talk about ..." Then I settle back into a relaxed but attentive posture and keep prompts and suggestions to a minimum. The idea here is to reverse the dynamism of the interaction by my taking the more passive role.

Some individuals relish the opportunity to expound on their issues, during which you can practice if necessary the redirection measures discussed above. But others will be sorely troubled by a relative absence of social cues, smile anxiously while confessing they don't know what to say and apologizing for it. As the resulting silence persists, both you and the other person will become increasingly uncomfortable.

There are two ways to deal with this. Sometimes I will make a soothing gesture, signaling they should try to relax, that everything is okay. Or I may explain what "we" hope to accomplish by this process, "Well you are accustomed to keeping people happy by saying what you think they want to hear. Actually I'm pretty happy with how things are going, so you don't have to worry about me. So here's an opportunity for you to figure out what might make you happy by paying attention to your needs, not someone else's ..." Prepare to have to repeat this redirection technique, since habitual pleasing is a lifetime (mal)adaptive maneuver. The idea is not to eradicate it—actually an impossibility—but to balance it with the potential to do the opposite now and then.

Finally, if with your support they are able to not only tolerate the process, but through it, reach into themselves to verbalize and clarify previously unexplored needs, you—cautiously of course—can recognize the achievement.

A Final Word on Reframing and Redirection

These examples of redirection are by no means exhaustive. Creativity and imagination are the only limits when it comes to developing redirection techniques to reinforce the learning that is the essence of effective counseling.

It is important to be measured in your redirection interventions. The wise coach does not always critique every misplayed ball or catch or shot. The same is true of the attentive therapist or counselor. In your role, you need to identify a single target disability and maintain focus on it. Then practice reframing and redirection whenever the individual you're working with becomes preoccupied with and distracted by subordinate concerns—which is routine when it comes to Attachment Disability. If you are patient and firm without being critical and the individual is cooperative, as their target problem starts to crumble, you will find that their other problems have a way of dissolving as well.

Your Takeaways

Clarification, *acceptance*, and *focus* are intertwined, not consecutive; inevitably your therapeutic work will be a mixture of all three.

▲

Reframing is *identifying* a target disability that is susceptible to change.

▲

Redirection is maintaining *focus* on the targeted disability.

▲

Identifying what can be changed includes its inverse: identifying what can't be changed ... today.

▲

Teach people to own their thoughts and feelings rather than hide from them.

▲

In a FUBAR world conflict-free options
are unlikely.

▲

Teach people to replace the word "should"
with the word "need."

▲

Crippling distrust is the primary
effect of trauma.

▲

Distrust is rarely liquidated by the direct
approach of earnestly soliciting trust.

▲

The most common cause of rambling and discursive speech is abandonment concerns.

▲

Always test your clarifying statements
by asking for feedback.

▲

Be concise and focused when making inquiries
and providing feedback.

▲

Recognize achievement without any subtext
that implies you expect continuing
performance.

▲

From time to time unstructure the dialogue
to give people a chance to focus on their own
needs rather their perception of yours.

▲

Undermine resistiveness by recognizing the
limits of your own powers.

▲

Habitual apologizing saps one's power.

▲

Redirect habitual apologizing by:
(1) gently recalling the counseling goal of asserting without apologizing
(2) restating without apologizing
(3) using a gesture during the session to flag the behavior
(4) providing a written prescription for posting to prompt recall

About the Author

Dr. Curran is a graduate of Saint Mary's University of Minnesota and Columbia College of Physicians and Surgeons. He completed a medical surgical internship at Saint Luke's Hospital in New York City and a psychiatric residency at the New York State Psychiatric Institute, also in New York. He is certified by the American Board of Psychiatry and Neurology. His books are based on fifty years' experience providing consulting services at state and private mental hospitals, county and private mental health centers, nursing homes, and residential treatment centers for adolescent sexual offenders and adult alcoholics, as well as a few years of clinical research and forty-four years of private practice.

Also by Dr. Curran:

Attachment Disability, Volume 1: The Hidden Cause of Adolescent Dysfunction and Lifelong Underperformance; Including a Plea for Psychiatric Diagnostic Reform

Trauma's lasting aftershock: misunderstood emotional disability

No one is immune from the pain of loss and abandonment. A beloved figure's death, a betrayal of trust, or abuse can inflict a degree of pain that is seriously traumatic. Those suffering such trauma may react with mistrust and depression, becoming unwilling or unable to reach out to others or accept attention and love. Their learning potential and life performance are impaired and their ability to develop stable relationships is disrupted: this is Attachment Disability.

Unfortunately, contemporary psychiatry minimizes the significance of trauma, leaving many attachment-disabled people misdiagnosed, mismanaged, and enduring unnecessary suffering.

In *Attachment Disability,* Dr. John Curran, a psychiatrist with decades of private and institutional practice, demonstrates that emotional disability is *always* trauma related. He draws on professional literature and dozens of case studies to define three types of Attachment Disability: Avoidant, Entangled, and Acting-Out. He persuasively advocates a psychiatric management style that avoids making things worse and helps people in pain clarify and accept their trauma and then focus on what they can change.

Dr. Curran concludes with suggestions on how American psychiatry can be invigorated by clearly distinguishing between mental illness and the emotional disability it generates.

Attachment Disability offers an invaluable contribution to the psychiatric profession and the people it seeks to serve.

> I wish I had this book thirty years ago; I would have made it required reading for every therapist on my staff.
> —Richard Obershaw, AMW, MSW, LICSW; author of the best-selling *Cry Until You Laugh: Comforting Guidance for Coping with Grief*

Price: $34.50
To order, contact:
Bidwell Learning Institute
8014 Olson Memorial Highway, Box 452
Golden Valley, MN 55427

www.ingramcontent.com/pod-product-compliance
Lightning Source LLC
Chambersburg PA
CBHW070929030426
42336CB00014BA/2599